The Effects of COVID-19 on Early Childhood Education

Research and Implications

By

Raquel Plotka and Ruth Guirguis

The Effects of COVID-19 on Early Childhood Education: Research and Implications

By Raquel Plotka and Ruth Guirguis

This book first published 2024

Ethics International Press Ltd, UK

British Library Cataloguing in Publication Data

A catalogue record for this book is available from the British Library

Print Book ISBN: 978-1-80441-304-3

eBook ISBN: 978-1-80441-305-0

Dedication

We would like to dedicate this book to essential early childhood professionals, who made our children feel safe during the darkest months of the pandemic.

Table of Contents

List of Tables and Figures

Preface

Raquel Plotka

This book, as many others, began with the need to find answers. In unprecedented times, we reach out to others for answers and when we don't find them, we reach inwards, exploring all the circles of our bio-ecological environment from the most proximal to the most distal. Some questions were pressed by our students, some by our own children, and many more by our racing minds. During the spring of 2020, there was very little information and guidance on how early childhood educators could support children and families. As social scholars, we used the only tools we had: research. We began looking for answers by posing research questions, collecting data in real-time as the crisis was evolving, and trying to generate some answers for ourselves and for our students.

So many of our students were working with young children in several capacities, and we wanted to give them the most useful information. Since little information was available at the time, we needed to start from the beginning, collecting data and developing instruments. Thus, some chapters of this book were written in the midst of the crisis. We were flying the plane while building it! These chapters include data collection and analysis. Some chapters were written later in the pandemic, with our ability to look back and reflect; because, by then, more research was available, these later chapters include literature reviews and present multiple voices, reflecting on experiences and lessons from different perspectives.

The most pressing questions during the first month of the pandemic were: what do we do next? How do we conduct early childhood education programs remotely? Is that even possible? Some of our students were developing curriculum and delivering materials door to door to children's homes. They turned to us for guidance asking questions like: What activities are more effective? What early childhood developmental learning goals can be addressed online? How do we engage families?

Families, children, and schools were experiencing stress, changes, and turmoil with educators at the center of this process, often negotiating on their own what to do next, how to implement curriculum, and how to keep young children engaged, calm, and reassured. We began with focus groups. The first few chapters emerged as answers for our students. With educators trying to cope with so much change at the most internal level, we asked how educators feel in their roles. What is their sense of efficacy in the middle of this crisis? The educators' voices were included to answer these questions.

Other questions emerged. For example, educators put together a curriculum and deliver lessons. Yet, something essential shifted. Children were seen only through a screen. What educators perceived to be effective through a screen did not always correlate with what parents were seeing at home. Educators began to ask, how are families experiencing these changes? In what ways do our experiences differ from those of the families who are seeing children face to face? Families' voices were included to answer these questions.

Teacher education programs shifted online, and even after the crisis came to a resolution, many programs have remained online. With so much focus on experiential learning in early childhood, we asked ourselves if it is possible to train early childhood educators remotely. We wondered, is this what our students want? The voices of our students, training to be teachers in the middle of a pandemic, were included as part of our answers.

As the pandemic evolved, more questions kept emerging, and we realized we needed diverse voices to address all these questions from multiple perspectives. For example, it became clear that socioeconomic status emerged as an indicator of how children and families fared. We also wondered about the experiences of immigrant children and their families.

During the spring of 2020, my one-year-old deaf nephew was waiting for his cochlear implant, but, because of the pandemic, there were delays in non-urgent procedures; as a result, his implant was delayed for several months. In addition, he was not getting any of the early intervention services that played a central role in his development. These interruptions were taking place during a prime stage for language development. We had to change plans. Instead of waiting for a cochlear implant, my family began taking sign language lessons so we could communicate with my nephew and foster language development throughout the months of the pandemic. This experience made me wonder about the experience of children with disabilities and their families, and we decided to include their voices in this book.

Furthermore, the value of early childhood educators is often overlooked. An especially overlooked group that played a key role during the pandemic is family child care providers. As the pandemic evolved, the rules, requirements, and regulations that providers had to follow and enforce kept changing, creating stress for educators, children, and families. We decided to also include the voices of this group in the book.

Several gaps in family policies in the U.S. became more visible during the pandemic. With children at home while parents worked remotely, it became harder to ignore that working parents have child care responsibilities. The U.S. had several challenges with work-family balance, especially when it came to child care support and universal access to early childhood education; the pandemic brought awareness to these challenges. Some of the lessons learned during this period should point toward minimizing inequalities in social support for families.

As the months mounted, we wondered what lessons we wanted to take for the future. Climate change, air quality issues, and other crises might arise that might bring about similar challenges as the ones brought about by COVID-19. This book summarizes the questions we asked, the answers we found, and the lessons we learned that might prove useful in the future.

It is my deepest hope that we never face similar challenges again. Nevertheless, resilience is the product of turning difficult experiences into lessons, and the collective experiences of COVID-19 should generate insightful recommendations and give us useful tools to face whatever new challenges the future might bring.

Ruth Guirguis

I walked into my 9:00 AM class on Wednesday, March 11, 2020. I began by reminding my pre-service teacher candidates that our entire course was on Blackboard and all the readings and assignments would continue to open every week. I took the first hour of class to answer any questions students had about the news on this virus going around in the city and what may happen in terms of our class. I explicitly remember telling them that if we were to shut down, our Blackboard modules were set for us to continue class remotely. I was not sure how or if that was actually the case, but I assured them we would finish the course somehow. The news was getting worse and far more frightening than one could imagine by the minute. Finally, on Friday, March 13th, 2020, I made the personal decision to no longer send my kids to school until we had more information. My kids at the time were all in our town's junior and senior high school and, at first, were excited about not having to go to school until further notice. Knowing they would be home gave me a superficial sense of safety and a drop of hope that this dire, seemingly apocalyptic situation would get better. Little did we know that what was ahead were months of lockdown and a rising death toll. We were petrified of leaving the house and avoided it at all costs.

Schools officially shut down on March 16th, and we were all introduced to an application called Zoom.

My kids attended classes on their laptops, and I taught and stared at a screen with black boxes for the remainder of the semester. There was so much chaos, panic, unknown, and desperation to return to normal. I tried to support my kids' learning as much as I could. I designated areas of the house for them to attend class and tried to implement a school schedule as much as possible; it was a struggle, especially for my youngest. She not only had a hard time learning through Zoom, but her anxiety skyrocketed. She had always been a sporty, social child who now had no outlet to manage her anxiety. Her attention to online lessons declined rapidly, and she quickly lost track of what was happening in each class and assignment deadlines. She was so behind that I decided to sit next to her during her most important classes to make sure she was paying attention and had to constantly redirect her focus. This added to her sense of frustration. I, too, was struggling with my own classes; trying to stay connected with my students and witnessing many of them miss classes and critical assignments was a feat in itself. My adult students were struggling as much as my own children.

Teaching and learning during COVID-19 were huge challenges. Those with access to technology and home support struggled less, but learning loss was a common variable for students at all levels. Months of online learning halted learning, and those who were falling behind were now in a critical situation. Young kids showed signs of anxiety and loneliness.

Trauma from isolation and home and food insecurities had severe negative effects on children's development. The amount of support students of all levels needed required educators and teacher preparation programs to revise their teaching and engagement protocols as our post-COVID students came in with very different learning needs and expectations. Reacquainting them with in-person learning was a challenge on its own. Learning to assess the needs of our new set of students was also a challenge that required educators to use research collected during this period and make decisions regarding curriculum that would help compensate for learning loss due to issues of inequality such as technology divides and gaps in special education services, physical care, and mental health supports. This book provides perspectives and data collected from different stakeholders during the COVID-19 pandemic. The purpose of this book is to provide lessons learned of what was effective during the pandemic, as well as the many systemic flaws of the United States educational system, to prepare all students for a better education.

Introduction
Early Childhood Education in the United States and COVID-19

The COVID-19 health crisis is an ongoing global pandemic that started in late 2019 and continues to affect people worldwide. The pandemic was caused by the emergence of a novel coronavirus known as SARS-CoV-2, which primarily spreads through respiratory droplets and symptoms ranging from mild to severe illness and led to an alarming number of fatalities. The pandemic has had a significant impact on various aspects of society (Xiang et al., 2021). Businesses and schools closed for extended periods of time, and people secluded themselves in their homes to remain safe as a race to develop a vaccine began. Business closures and massive layoffs, along with disruptions to supply chains, posed a major strain in the United States and worldwide economies.

COVID-19 has had a significant impact on early childhood education in the U.S. and worldwide. In the U.S. the early childhood education (ECE) field has historically operated on slim resources with regard to wages and low public funding; during the pandemic this weak infrastructure became evident (Kim et al., 2022). The early childhood education system in the U.S. is highly fragmented and is characterized by a combination of public and private providers, various funding sources, and a lack of a unified national framework. The pandemic had several impacts on this already fragile system.

The Central Role of Early Childhood Education

The importance of early childhood education has been widely established in the literature. Research on quality early childhood education has consistently demonstrated its significant and positive impact on various aspects of a child's life and development (e.g.,

Burchinal et al., 2000; National Institute of Child Health and Human Development Early Child Care Research Network, 2000). The early years of a child's life are a period of rapid brain development, and quality ECE programs have been shown to provide stimulating and nurturing environments that support cognitive development, language acquisition, and the formation of neural connections crucial for future learning.

Quality programs support a child's social skills and emotional development. Through interactions with qualified professionals and other children, children learn how to interact positively with peers, manage their emotions, and develop empathy, self-regulation, and conflict-resolution skills, which are critical for success in school and life.

Similarly, high-quality ECE contributes to better cognitive development, including improved grades, language skills, and problem-solving abilities (Burchinal et al., 2000). Early childhood education experiences have been shown to build a strong academic foundation for children before they enter formal education systems. Children who participated in ECE have been found to develop early literacy and math skills, narrative and language skills, and the ability to cope with social demands (Barnett et al., 1995; National Institute of Child Health and Human Development Early Child Care Research Network, 2000).

Similarly, access to high-quality early education has been found to help reduce achievement gaps due to socioeconomic disparities, and children from low socioeconomic backgrounds often benefit the most from ECE programs. In addition, participation in ECE has been shown to reduce special education needs later in life, as identifying and addressing learning disabilities early often reduces developmental delays and the need for special education services in later years (Kagan & Kauerz, 2015).

Research on the long-term effects of quality ECE has consistently demonstrated its significant and positive impact on various aspects of a child's life and development. For example, children who participated in high-quality ECE programs were more likely to graduate from high school, pursue higher education, and earn higher levels of education compared to those who did not attend such programs (McCoy et al., 2017). Consequently, adults who attended high-quality ECE programs in the past tend to have higher earnings in their careers, which benefit both the adults and the entire economy (Ruhm & Waldfogel, 2012). Finally, long-term studies have shown that individuals who participated in quality ECE programs are less likely to need welfare assistance or to engage in criminal activities, saving society monetary and societal costs (Yoshikawa, 1995).

Early Childhood Education Systems in the U.S.

Despite the importance of quality early childhood education, the ECE field in the U.S. is largely underfunded and fractured with variations in access and affordability. Early childhood education in the United States is a complex system that encompasses a wide range of programs and services designed to support the development of young children from birth to age eight. The system is characterized by a combination of public and private providers, various funding sources, and a lack of a unified national framework (Kagan & Kauerz, 2015). Some key components of the early childhood system in the U.S. include state pre-kindergarten programs, special education and early intervention services for young children with disabilities, child care and home-based programs, family-based centers, private preschools, and public kindergartens in public schools.

Many states have their own pre-kindergarten (pre-K) programs that offer early education services to 3-4-year-old children. The quality, funding, and availability of these programs vary by state (Kagan & Kauerz, 2015). On the other hand, programs such as Head Start and Early Head Start are federal programs and provide comprehensive early childhood education, health, nutrition, and parent involvement services to low-income children and their families from birth to age five. Child care centers and home-based family centers play a central role in providing early education to young children. Private and public child care centers and home-based child care providers offer services for infants, toddlers, and preschool-aged children. Low-income families are often eligible for child care subsidies to help cover the cost of child care services. Public school systems offer kindergarten programs for 5-year-olds, and some districts also provide pre-kindergarten programs (Kagan & Kauerz, 2015). At the same time, many families rely on private preschools and early learning centers exist throughout the country to serve children from infancy through preschool age. Special Education Services and early intervention services are available for children with delays and disabilities, starting from a very young age. These services are often provided through public school districts and through home visiting programs.

The early childhood education system in the United States is diverse and varies significantly from state to state in terms of quality, availability, and funding. Additionally, there is ongoing debate and advocacy for increased investment in early childhood education to improve access and quality, as research suggests that quality early education can have a significant impact on a child's long-term development and educational success (Kagan & Kauerz, 2015). The qualifications and compensation for ECE educators vary by type of setting, and the terms teacher, educator, ECE professional, and caregiver are often used interchangeably to describe similar roles.

Early Childhood Education and COVID-19

COVID-19 has had a significant impact on early childhood education in the U.S. and worldwide. In the U.S. the ECE field has historically operated on slim resources with regard to wages and low public funding; this weak infrastructure became evident during the pandemic (Kim et al., 2022). This had negative impacts on children, educators, families, and teacher preparation programs. Some of the negative impacts included mental health concerns, social and emotional delays, limited access to healthcare, substantial learning loss, lack of school professional services, and housing and food instabilities.

The pandemic forced many early childhood education programs, including preschools and daycare centers, to close, implement online learning, or incorporate strict safety measures to prevent the spread of the virus. These disruptions resulted in short and long-term effects for children, families, and educators (Kim et al., 2022).

For children, the disruptions caused by the many phases of the pandemic have had impacts on cognitive, social, and emotional development. With the closure of learning centers and the limited opportunities for face-to-face interaction, many young children missed out on critical learning opportunities. Early childhood is a crucial period of social development and the lack of continuous social interactions with teachers or peers might hinder children's development of social skills and emotional intelligence. At the same time, the pandemic has forced parents and other family members to take a more significant role in their children's education and development while balancing work and other responsibilities.

The pandemic exacerbated existing inequalities in early childhood education in the U.S. Children from lower socioeconomic (SES) status faced greater challenges in continuing their education during lockdowns, as access to technology and/or in-person learning opportunities varied extensively across different SES levels.

Educational institutions, educators, and policymakers have tried to address these challenges by implementing distance learning initiatives and creating safe environments for children to learn. Several lessons were learned through these trial and error attempts, and this book attempted to gather the lessons learned through the pandemic in order to generate implications for the future. Climate change, air quality issues, and other crises might arise that might bring about similar challenges as the ones brought about by COVID-19. This book summarizes the questions asked, the answers generated, and the lessons learned that might prove useful in the future.

Organization of this Book

This book is organized in three sections. The first section consists of original research conducted during the first months of the pandemic. These studies were developed to inform practices throughout the months of the pandemic and are focused on experiences with virtual learning.

The second section consists of a combination of literature reviews and original research illustrating the way the pandemic has had different effects on diverse populations. These chapters were written later on during the pandemic, when more information regarding the impacts of COVID-19 became available. For this section, the authors collaborated with contributors with specialized expertise.

Lastly, the final section constitutes a reflection on the changes the pandemic has had on the ECE profession and on the lessons learned and implications for ECE policy to ensure a better future.

References

Barnett, W. S. (1995). Long-term effects of early childhood programs on cognitive and school outcomes. *The future of children*, 25-50.

Burchinal, M.R., Roberts, J.E., Riggins Jr, R., Zeisel, S., Neebe, E., & Bryant, D. (2000). Relating quality of center-based child care to early cognitive and language development longitudinally. *Child Development, 71*(2), 339–357.

Kagan, L., & Kauerz, K. (2015). *Early childhood systems: Transforming early learning*. Teachers College Press.

Kim, Y., Montoya, E., Doocy, S., Austin, L., & Whitebook, M. (2022). Impacts of COVID-19 on the early care and education sector in California: Variations across program types. *Early Childhood Research Quarterly (60)*, 348-362.

National Institute of Child Health and Human Development Early Child Care Research Network (2000). The relation of child care to cognitive and language development. *Child Development, 71*(4), 960–980.

McCoy, D. C., Yoshikawa, H., Ziol-Guest, K. M., Duncan, G. J., Schindler, H. S., Magnuson, K., & Shonkoff, J. P. (2017). Impacts of early childhood education on medium-and long-term educational outcomes. *Educational Researcher, 46*(8), 474-487.

Ruhm, C., & Waldfogel, J. (2012). Long-term effects of early childhood care and education. *Nordic Economic Policy Review, 1*(1), 23-51.

Xiang, S., Rasool, S., Hang, Y., Javid, K., Javed, T., & Artene, A. E. (2021). The Effect of COVID-19 Pandemic on Service Sector Sustainability and Growth. *Frontiers in psychology, 12*, 633597. https://doi.org/10.3389/fpsyg.2021.633597

Yoshikawa, H. (1995). Long-term effects of early childhood programs on social outcomes and delinquency. *The future of children*, 51-75.

Section I

Research on the Effects of COVID-19 on Teachers, Families, and Teacher Preparation Programs

Chapter 1
COVID-19, Virtual Learning, and Early Childhood Educators' Experiences

During the spring months of 2020, most early childhood education (ECE) programs in the United States and around the world moved to online instructional platforms. Early childhood educators were faced with teaching fully remote programs with little to no preparation time. This drastic change in instruction, along with limited teaching resources, as well as finite school and family support, created a unique demand on teachers' abilities to deliver instruction. Many early childhood programs attempted to initiate support systems to meet the needs of their teachers and students. Yet, there was no uniform call regarding what those supports should have been. Hence, teacher experiences varied widely (Pattnaik & Jalongo, 2022).

Teaching remotely presented a challenge to all educators, as well as faculty at the undergraduate and graduate levels (Kim, 2020; Plotka & Guirguis, 2020). Specifically, remote teaching in the early childhood grades created a unique set of challenges due to the active nature of young children's learning; these challenges directly impacted the engagement of young children in meaningful learning experiences. Yet, very little is currently known about teachers' experiences and the challenges they faced while adjusting to this new reality. Nor is much yet known about which of the different strategies teachers used to engage children were found to be most effective. Furthermore, there has been a paucity of research exploring the impact these challenges support systems have had on teachers' sense of self-efficacy during this health crisis.

According to Eadie et al. (2022), there were adverse consequences to the ECE workforce as well as to the well-being of early childhood educators. Specifically, a teacher's sense of self-efficacy has been shown to play a key role in children's academic and behavioral outcomes in the preschool classroom (Gebbie et al., 2011). The present study aimed at exploring early childhood teachers' experiences with teaching virtually during unprecedented times, the challenges teachers experienced, the support teachers may have had or may have needed, and the impact these elements had on their respective sense of self-efficacy.

Early Childhood Educators' Challenges While Teaching Online

Most early childhood educators subscribe to the assumption that learning is an active process fostered by an environment that provides opportunities for exploration, manipulation, social interactions, and play (Plotka & Guirguis, 2020). These assumptions are rooted in the works of theorists such as Piaget and Vygotsky, as well as the most important approaches in early childhood education, such as those of Montessori or Reggio Emilia (Dodd-Nufrio, 2011; Edwards, 2002). In particular, Piaget believed that children are active learners and create knowledge by exploration and manipulation; children progress from manipulating objects to the ability to manipulate symbols (Piaget, 1932). Similarly, Vygotsky believed that young children make meaning of the world through social interactions with peers and adults (Vygotsky, 1978). Following these theorists, most approaches in early childhood education incorporate exploration through play, music, and the arts (Dodd-Nufrio, 2011). Thus, the idea of providing instruction to young children through a screen is mostly foreign to early childhood education and, for the most part, does not adequately align with theoretical and practical frameworks (Plotka & Guirguis, 2020); this made the transition to online teaching especially challenging for many early childhood teachers.

It should be noted, however, that even before the COVID-19 health crisis, online and virtual instruction had been expanding both in the United States and globally. For example, the Upstart program has been providing online preschool instruction for thousands of children in the

United States since 2013 (Mader, 2018). The program, funded by the federal government, has delivered online instruction to preschool children in Idaho, Mississippi, Indiana, South Carolina, rural Ohio, and Philadelphia. Thirty percent of young children in Utah attend this online preschool program (Mader, 2018). In addition, though there is currently little research on the academic results of Upstart, there is a limited body of research exploring the challenges teachers (mostly those outside the United States) have faced while teaching young children online during COVID.

The existing studies point to challenges in implementing curriculum in a developmentally appropriate way. For example, early childhood educators in Turkey reported trouble with remote learning due to a lack of student engagement and motivation (Korkmaz & Toraman, 2020). Another concern early childhood educators reported was the lack of authentic strategies provided to modify instruction and meet different types of learning styles virtually. The use of social interaction, group work, small group pair and share, and many other typical peer and collaborative teaching strategies was challenging, especially at the beginning of the new remote learning world (Korkmaz & Toraman, 2020). Keeping young children engaged in online learning proved to be the most difficult task for teachers (Szente, 2020). Particularly difficult was the task of having to reduce the time spent on a given topic to maintain students' attention and engagement while also embedding storytime, songs, music, and movement in a fluid and consistent way throughout the lesson. Teachers also navigated ways to have students share their thoughts more frequently so that teachers could hear thoughts and ideas from all students.

Pre-pandemic studies showed that some online activities allow for social interaction between students while they practice turn-taking, conversational language, and social etiquette (Theodotou & Kulovana, 2012). Similarly, studies have shown that young children benefit from adult assistance while engaging in remote learning (Theodotou & Kulovana, 2012). Teachers tried certain strategies to engage children in remote learning with social interactions, and they had some successes. Since, for example, the virtual learning environment encourages turn-taking when individuals in online classes speak, teachers are able to hear and respond to students more effectively than in a typical in-person learning environment (Szente, 2020). Nevertheless, there has not been much more exploration of the types of activities that teachers found most effective while teaching online or to what degree early childhood teachers felt they were effective at virtually facilitating social interactions with young children.

Lastly, early childhood educators reported the challenges they experienced in managing students' emotional well-being. The adverse effect of a drastic change in routines, including separation from peers and teachers, has impacted young children's emotional and social development (Singh et al., 2020). Young children have displayed feelings of irritability, uncertainty, fear, and isolation (Singh et al., 2020). While teachers typically gather information about children's well-being using a variety of methods, including observation of children's play, interactions, and drawings, the online platform can present a challenge for teachers in observing and understanding children's well-being. Little has been explored about teachers' experiences or their ability to assess well-being in young children and their perceptions of children's emotional states.

Teacher Sense of Self-Efficacy

A teacher's sense of self-efficacy has been shown to play a key role in children's academic and behavioral outcomes in the preschool classroom (Gebbie et al., 2011). Self-efficacy is described as a person's belief in their ability to succeed in a specific situation (Bandura, 1997). Bandura explained that these beliefs determined how people feel, think, and act; he proposed that a sense of self-efficacy affects a person's perseverance in overcoming challenges, the level of effort they apply, and their presence (Bandura, 1997). Teachers' sense of self-efficacy is the belief teachers have in their ability to organize the necessary activities to engage children in learning and impact student development and achievement. Promoting student learning involves a teacher's ability to create and plan developmentally meaningful activities, openly communicate with and support families, and assess and manage behaviors (Skaalvik & Skaalvik, 2010). Additionally, it constitutes the teacher's belief in their ability to manage teaching tasks, obligations, and challenges (Barni et al., 2019). High levels of self-efficacy in teachers have been related to high levels of self-esteem, job satisfaction, and motivation (Pinchevsky & Bogler, 2014), as well as children's academic success and positive behavioral outcomes (Gebbie et al., 2011). Yet the degree to which early childhood teachers felt self-efficacy while teaching remotely during COVID has not been explored.

Influence of Support Systems on Teacher Self-Efficacy

Teachers' sense of self-efficacy can prove especially important during times of crisis. Despite the many challenges educators face while teaching online, a teacher's sense of self-efficacy is positively correlated to the support they receive from both administration and parents (Stipek, 2012). According to Stipek (2012), administrators play a key role in a teacher's sense of self-efficacy; support from school administration could improve teacher self-efficacy, whereas a lack thereof could hinder it. Teachers' perception of support from their administrators has been shown to have a direct relationship with student performance (Stipek, 2012). Similarly, Wahlstrom and Louis (2008) found that a teacher's perception of support from their leadership had a direct effect on instructional practices. In a study surveying teachers in Turkey, teachers expressed that one of their biggest challenges in shifting to online instruction was negative attitudes between the administration and teachers, as well as a lack of support from the school administration (Korkmaz & Toraman, 2020).

Similarly, according to Skaalvik and Skaalvik (2010), teachers' perceptions of parental support were found to be as critical to teachers' sense of efficacy as administrative support; teachers' perceptions of their relationships with families were associated with higher self-efficacy levels (Skaalvik & Skaalvik, 2010). Specifically, self-efficacy was found to be influenced by ongoing communication and collaborative relationships between parents and teachers (Skaalvik & Skaalvik, 2010). The online learning environment can prove challenging for communication between teachers and families (Leonhardt, 2020). But it also can create opportunities for communication; in some ways, communication might have increased during this time. In a Norwegian school district study, communication between parents and teachers increased during the pandemic. Parents were able to connect with their children's struggles and challenges with learning because they were able to see it with their own eyes in their homes and daily lives. Parents taking on the role of in-home educators allowed them to be more understanding and strive to communicate with their child's teacher more often than during a typical in-person school day (Bubb & Jones, 2020). Nevertheless, this study was conducted in an elementary school, and it is unclear how increased parent participation in their children's learning might have affected the virtual preschool setting, where communication with families is even more central.

The Present Study

The COVID-19 health crisis, and the resulting expansion of online instruction in the United States and the world, both have presented the opportunity to study the underexplored area of experiences and challenges related to online teaching in early childhood. Given the central role teacher self-efficacy plays in teacher motivation and children's behavioral and academic outcomes, this study aimed to explore teacher self-efficacy among those teaching online during the COVID-19 pandemic. This study especially aimed at examining challenges and supports that teachers experienced during this period, specifically teacher perception of support from the school administration, support from parents, and increases in teacher-parent communication. Finally, the role of these support systems in teachers' sense of self-efficacy during the COVID-19 pandemic was also explored. The present study aimed to answer the following questions:

1. What have been teachers' most common experiences and challenges while teaching young children online during the COVID-19 pandemic?
2. Has teaching online during the pandemic impacted teachers' sense of self-efficacy?
3. To what extent has support from the school administration, support from families, and open communication with families impacted teacher self-efficacy during the COVID-19 pandemic?

Method

Participants

Participants were 54 preschool teachers who were teaching young children online due to the COVID-19 health crisis in a central metropolitan area in the U.S. Teachers worked in a variety of early childhood education settings, such as early childhood programs and private preschools. Table 1.1 describes the participants and shows the frequency and percentages of the participants' respective titles and the type of early childhood education program in which they taught. Most participants held the title of teacher (n = 37, 69.8%). The largest number of participants indicated working in child care programs (n = 15, 30.6%), followed by private preschools (n= 9, 18.4%). One individual did not provide informed consent, and this individual's data were removed from the dataset, thereby reducing the final sample size to 53. Participants described their classroom composition. The ages of the children in their classes ranged from 17 months old to 9 years of age, with a mean of 4.16 (SD = 1.52). The number of children in the classes ranged from 8 to 30, with a mean of 15.04 children (SD = 4.32).

Survey Item	n	%
Title		
Teacher	37	69.8
Assistant Teacher	16	30.2
Total	53	100.0
School Description		
Public School	5	10.2
Private Preschool	9	18.4
Private Faith-Based/Parochial	6	12.2
Head Start	3	6.1
Universal Pre-K	8	16.3
Child Care Program	15	30.6
Other publicly funded preschool program	3	6.1
Total	49	100.0

Table 1.1 *Participant Demographics*

Procedure and Instrument

This was a convenience sample made up of early childhood education teachers. Teachers were asked to fill out an online survey about their experiences teaching young children online during the COVID-19 crisis. Educators teaching young children solely online were recruited to fill out the survey after institutional review approval was obtained. Data collection took place a few months into the pandemic in the spring and summer of 2020. Teachers were recruited by word of mouth and volunteered to participate in the study. To answer the research questions, a survey was sent to early childhood teachers to measure their teaching experiences, challenges, and sense of self-efficacy. Teacher reports have been widely used in the study of social processes in the classrooms and teacher self-efficacy (Rimm-Kaufman et al., 2000) and have been shown to have predictive validity (Fuhs et al., 2015). The survey consisted of quantitative data, and participants reported their experiences at a single point in time. Before the survey was administered, it was shared with small focus groups of preschool teachers teaching online to ensure that it reflected common experiences and processes taking place in the classroom based on teachers' experiences. The survey consisted of a four-point scale ranging from 1 (not effective), 2 (somewhat effective), 3 (effective), and 4 (very effective). Item descriptions for the survey are provided in the Results section. The survey assessed the following constructs:

Teacher Experiences

Several survey questions were designed to get a well-rounded sense of teachers' experiences and challenges. One of the questions asked teachers to rate items related to teachers' challenges in supporting children's development and skills virtually. Teachers were also asked to rate the developmentally appropriate activities that they found most effective when teaching online and to assess the level of children's participation in virtual learning activities. Lastly, one of the questions was designed to measure teachers' perceptions of children's well-being.

Teachers' Sense of Self-Efficacy

Teachers were asked to report on their sense of self-efficacy before the pandemic while teaching in-person and again during the pandemic while teaching online. The items touching on teacher self-efficacy were adapted from the teacher self-efficacy early childhood survey developed by Epstein and Willhite (2017).

Teachers' Perception of Support

Teachers were asked to report on their experiences of support from their school administration. It was also requested that teachers rate the level of support they perceived themselves as receiving from families in their program. Lastly, teachers were asked about the level of communication with families during remote learning.

Results

This study aimed to explore teachers' experiences and challenges while they taught online during the COVID-19 pandemic and the role these experiences, as well as their perceptions of support from administrators and parents, played in their sense of self-efficacy.

Research Question 1: What Have Been the Most Common Teacher Experiences and Challenges?

The first research question aimed at exploring teachers' challenges and experiences during the pandemic while they taught young children online. To answer this question, descriptive statistics were used to illustrate the extent of teacher experiences. The results in Table 1.2 show that teachers found it challenging to adequately address each of these early childhood goals through virtual modes of teaching. Teachers found it most challenging to support social skills, such as helping children make friends, adjust to routines, and follow rules. Teachers experienced fewer challenges when it came to teaching academic content and skills.

How challenging was it to address each of the following early childhood education goals when teaching online?	N	Min	Max	M	SD
Supporting family needs	53	1	4	2.05	0.86
Helping children learn the alphabet, numbers, or other information that will prepare them for school	53	1	4	2.32	0.93
Helping children make friends	53	1	4	2.98	0.99
Helping children interact with other children positively	53	1	4	2.45	0.95
Giving children the opportunity to play	53	1	4	2.45	1.06
Helping children learn how to follow rules	53	1	4	2.6	0.96
Helping children learn about appropriate behaviors	53	1	4	2.57	0.88

How challenging was it to address each of the following early childhood education goals when teaching online?	N	Min	Max	M	SD
Helping children learn about classrooms routines and schedules so they are prepared for school	53	1	4	2.87	1.05

Table 1.2 *Teachers' Experiences of Challenges*

Implementing activities that were developmentally appropriate and engaging for children was reported to be one of the most challenging aspects of teaching young children online. Teachers found that not all strategies worked equally effectively. Table 1.3 shows that teachers rated storytime/reading books, games and social activities, sing-alongs, and one-on-one time between children and teachers as the most effective activities on the online platform. Direct instruction and hands-on activities without an adult assisting at home were the least effective.

Teachers tried different online activities to engage children during this time. What activities were most effective?	N	Min	Max	M	SD
Storytime/reading books	53	1	4	3.05	0.86
Games and social activities	53	1	4	3.07	0.89
Direct instruction	53	1	4	2.39	0.81
Sing-alongs	53	1	4	3.05	0.79
One-on-one time with teachers	53	1	4	3.13	0.83
Hands-on activities with an adult assisting	53	1	4	2.94	0.94
Hands-on activities without an adult assisting	53	1	4	1.96	0.8
Art activities	53	1	4	2.7	0.93

Table 1.3 *Activities Teachers Found Effective*

Teachers reported that many children did not participate in several of the online learning activities designed to engage them. For example, Table 1.4 shows that the largest number of teachers indicated that only about half the class typically participated in group activities (n = 18, 34%).

How many children typically participated in learning activities?	N	%
None	2	3.8
A few children	15	28.3
About half of class	18	34.0
Almost the whole class	14	26.4
Total	53	100

Table 1.4 *Children's Participation in Online Learning Activities*

Managing students' emotional well-being was reported as a major challenge for early childhood educators. The negative effect of the sudden and significant changes in younger children's routines, including their separation from teachers and friends, has impacted their emotional and social development (Singh et al., 2020). In the present study, and through the survey provided to teachers, 53 early childhood teachers were asked using a four-point scale ranging from 1 (not at all), 2 (somewhat), 3 (moderately), and 4 (extremely) to rate their perception of the emotions their students felt during remote learning. Teachers reported that 44% of the students were somewhat disengaged, while 36% were very disengaged. Results showed that 44% of students were somewhat confused, 44% were very confused, 50% of students were somewhat overwhelmed, and 25% were very overwhelmed. Teachers also reported that 45% of the students were somewhat sad, 25% of them were very sad, 28% were somewhat anxious, 61% of the students were very anxious, 36% felt somewhat lonely, 24% felt very lonely, and 39% were somewhat scared, while 21% were very scared. In addition, Table 1.5 shows teachers' perceptions of children's emotions.

Emotions Young Children Experience During Online Classes	N	Min	Max	M	SD
Confusion	53	1.00	4.00	2.67	0.95
Disengagement	53	1.00	4.00	2.56	0.86
Loneliness	53	1.00	4.00	2.03	0.97
Fear	53	1.00	4.00	1.86	0.94
Sadness	53	1.00	4.00	2.18	0.89
Overwhelmingness	53	1.00	4.00	2.18	0.85
Anxiousness	53	1.00	4.00	2.28	0.94

Table 1.5 *Teachers' Perceptions of Children's Well-Being*

Research Question 2: Has Teaching Online During the Pandemic Impacted Teachers' Sense of Self-Efficacy?

To address this research question, the researchers created two measures of teacher efficacy. One measure reflected the efficacy of teachers before the onset of the pandemic while they were teaching in person, and the second measure reflected teacher efficacy after the onset of the pandemic. Based on the small sample size and unequal variances, paired t-tests were used to assess teacher efficacy before the COVID-19 pandemic, while teachers taught in person, and during the COVID-19 crisis, while they taught online (Carifio & Perla, 2009; de Winter & Dodou, 2010; Guerra et al., 2016; Norman, 2010). Table 1.6 shows that teachers experienced significantly lower levels of self-efficacy while teaching online after the onset of the COVID-19 pandemic than before the pandemic when they taught in person. All items in the self-efficacy measure were statistically significant, which indicates that teachers felt a significantly lower sense of self-efficacy when teaching remotely during the pandemic; this decline was consistent among all aspects of self-efficacy.

Question	Mean Pre Pandemic	Mean Post Pandemic	t	p
How much can you do to control disruptive behavior in the classroom?	3.45	1.94	11.78	0.001
How much can you do to motivate students who show low interest in learning activities?	3.52	2.13	11.22	0.001
How much can you do to get students to believe they can do well in school?	3.69	2.60	8.24	0.001
How much can you do to help your students value learning?	3.54	2.60	8.92	0.001
How much can you do to get children to follow classroom rules?	3.58	2.16	11.34	0.001
How much can you do to calm a student who is disruptive or noisy?	3.33	1.96	11.34	0.001
To what extent can you craft good questions for your students?	3.39	2.96	3.96	0.001
How well can you establish a classroom management system with each group of students?	3.58	2.43	10.24	0.001
How much can you use a variety of assessment strategies?	3.41	2.58	6.30	0.001
To what extent can you provide an alternative explanation as an example when students are confused?	3.56	2.56	7.42	0.001
How much can you assist families in helping their children do well in school?	3.35	2.88	5.14	0.001

Table 1.6 *Paired Samples T-Tests Comparing Teachers' Self-Efficacy (n=53)*

Research Question 3: To What Extent Did Experiencing Support Predict Teacher Self-Efficacy During the COVID-19 Pandemic?

To answer this research question, the individual items were averaged to arrive at a composite score. These composite scores were computed so that simultaneous multiple linear regression could be conducted, predicting teacher self-efficacy. The efficacy scale used in this study was previously validated using all 24 items (long version) as well as using only 12 items (short version) from the scale (Tschannen-Moran & Hoy, 2001). The long version of the scale has a Cronbach's alpha of .94 and the short version of the scale has a Cronbach's alpha of .90. Tschannen-Moran and Hoy (2000) also conducted an EFA on each subscale of the instrument: instructional strategies, management, and engagement. All three subscales, for both the long and short versions, have Cronbach alphas ranging from .81-.90. Therefore, for this study, a composite of the scores obtained from the short teacher self-efficacy scale version before the onset of the COVID-19 pandemic was used. Scores ranged from 2.62 to 4.00, with an average score of 3.50 (SD = 0.40) (Epstein & Willhite, 2015; Tschannen-Moran & Hoy, 2001). Composite teacher self-efficacy scores after the onset of the COVID-19 pandemic ranged from 1.00 to 4.00, with an average score of 2.46 (SD = 0.60). The composites were also reliable, with Cronbach's alphas ranging from .90 for the pre-COVID-19 teacher self-efficacy composite to .91 for the post-COVID-19 teacher self-efficacy composite.

Research question 3 asked to what extent support from school administration, support from schools in the program, and open communication with families predicted teacher efficacy after the onset of the COVID-19 pandemic. To address this research question, simultaneous multiple linear regression procedures were conducted. Support from school administration, support from families in the program, and open communication with families were entered as predictors in the model. Prior to interpreting the regression model, tolerance and the variance inflation factors (VIF) were examined. Per Cohen et al. (2004), the results indicated that multicollinearity was not an issue, given that tolerance values were above .10 and VIF values were less than 10.

The model was statistically significant (F(3, 49) = 4.41, p < .01, R2 = .165.) and accounted for 16.5% of the variance in teacher efficacy after the onset of the COVID-19 pandemic. The findings in Table 1.7 revealed that an increase in feeling supported by the families in the program significantly predicted teacher efficacy after the onset of the COVID-19 pandemic (β = .24, p = .04). Feeling supported by the school administration and keeping open communication with families were not statistically significant in the model.

Model	*B*	*SE*	*β*	*t*	*p*	Tol.	VIF
I feel supported by the school administration.	0.16	0.10	0.21	1.50	0.13	0.81	1.23
I feel supported by the families in the program.	0.24	0.11	0.31	2.11	0.04	0.72	1.37
I was able to keep open communication with families.	0.03	0.13	0.03	0.24	0.81	0.76	1.30

Table 1.7 *Regression Coefficients Predicting Teachers' Self-Efficacy*

Note. TOL = tolerance, VIF = Variance Inflation Factor. Overall model (F(3, 49) = 4.41, $p = .008$, $R^2 = .165$.

Discussion

The COVID-19 health crisis has forced many early childhood education programs in the United States and around the world to shift to online instruction. This situation has presented the opportunity to study the experiences and challenges teachers of young children face while teaching online. Despite the global shift to online teaching, very few studies have explored early childhood educators' experiences and challenges. The present study attempted to bridge this gap in knowledge by addressing the experiences and challenges teachers faced. Similarly, despite the central role of teachers' sense of self-efficacy in children's developmental outcomes, no study has assessed the role of online teaching in teachers' sense of self-efficacy. Lastly, this study attempted to study the role of support systems in teachers' experience of self-efficacy. Online education has been growing in recent years, and it is expected to continue to grow even after the COVID-19 health crisis is resolved. The lessons learned throughout his period can inform future online practices for teaching very young children.

Major Findings

One of the major findings of this study indicates that teachers experienced challenges when attempting to address early childhood goals in the virtual setting. Teachers found that supporting social skills, such as helping children make friends, adjust to routines, and follow rules was especially challenging. They also reported that teaching academic content and skills was less difficult. Implementing developmentally appropriate activities was also challenging in the virtual setting. Nevertheless, teachers found storytime/reading books, games, social activities, sing-alongs, and one-on-one time between children and teachers to be most effective. Hands-on activities were only effective when adults were able to assist the children at home. Direct instruction and hands-on activities without an adult assisting at home were not very effective. However, children's participation and engagement suffered, as many teachers reported that several children did not participate in many of the learning activities. Lastly, teachers found that they perceived children as having experienced mostly confusion, disengagement, and loneliness during this period.

The pandemic and the need to teach online have significantly affected teachers' sense of self-efficacy. Teachers reported that their confidence declined when it came to their ability to control disruptive behavior, motivate students, and help children believe in themselves and value learning. Similarly, teachers felt a decline in confidence in their ability to help children follow rules, calm disruptive children, craft good questions, establish classroom management systems, use a variety of assessment strategies, clarify information to confused children, and help families. Despite these challenges and the decrease in teachers' sense of self-efficacy, however, teachers revealed that feeling supported by the families in the program significantly impacted their levels of self-efficacy.

Lessons Learned and Implications for the Future

One of the most important lessons learned from this study was that when preschool teaching went online, children's social skills suffered the most. While teachers felt that helping children develop social skills, follow rules, or adjust to routines was extremely difficult, they found teaching academic content less challenging. This finding should be considered highly informative when contemplating online education platforms for young children, as academic skills might be promoted at the expense of social skills.

This study showed that teachers have tried to engage young children in activities that are best translated to an online platform. The activities that teachers found most effective, such as story-time and sing-alongs, were teacher-centered. Online platforms do not seem to easily incorporate child-centered activities, such as exploration and self-expression. Furthermore, despite teachers' great efforts, almost half of their students did not participate in such activities, pointing to the challenges in engaging young children in online learning.

Lastly, responses to the survey discussed here show that teaching online during a pandemic has affected teachers' sense of self-efficacy. The most important sources of support that teachers received came from families in their programs. This finding should be considered when designing interventions to promote teachers' sense of self-efficacy during crises. Administrators should look into expanding opportunities for teacher-family support. In addition, since teachers felt their greatest sources of support came from families, administrators should look into providing consistent sources of support for teachers during major shifts and crises. In sum, the pandemic has presented the opportunity to learn what has worked and what has not when teaching young children online. It also revealed the need to provide teachers with more sources of support to promote teachers' sense of self-efficacy.

References

Bandura, A. (1997). *Self-efficacy: The exercise of control.* Henry Holt & Co. New York, NY.

Barni, D., Danioni, F., & Benevene, P. (2019). Teachers' self-efficacy: The role of personal values and motivations for teaching. *Frontiers in Psychology, 10,* 1645.https://doi.org/10.3389/fpsyg.2019.01645.

Bubb, S. & Jones, M-A. (2020). Learning from the COVID-19 home-schooling experience: Listening to pupils, parents/caregivers, and teachers. Sage.

Carifio, J. & Perla, R. (2009). Resolving the 50-year Debate Around using and Misusing Likert Scales. *Medical education, 42,* 1150-2. https://onlinelibrary.wiley.com/doi/abs/10.1111/j.1365-2923.2008.03172.x.

Cohen, J. C., Aiken, L. S., & West, S. G. (2004). Regression analysis for the behavioral sciences. Newbury Park, CA: Sage.

De Winter, J.C.F. and Dodou D. (2010). Five-Point Likert Items: t test versus Mann-Whitney-Wilcoxon, Practical Assessment, Research and Evaluation, 15(11). https://doi.org/10.7275/bj1p- ts64.

Dodd-Nufrio, A. T. (2011, October 1). Reggio Emilia, Maria Montessori, and John Dewey: Dispelling teachers' misconceptions and understanding theoretical foundations. ttps://www.researchgate.net/publication/226689076_Reggio_Emilia_Maria_Montessori_and_John_Dewey_Dispelling_Teachers'_Misconceptions_and_Understanding_Theoretical_Foundations

Eadie, P., Levickis, P., Murray, L., Page, J., Elek, C., & Church, A. (2021b). Early childhood educators' well-being during the COVID-19 pandemic. *Early Childhood Education Journal, 49*(5), 903–913. https://doi.org/10.1007/s10643-021-01203-3

Edwards, C. P. (2002). Three approaches from Europe: Waldorf, Montessori and Reggio Emilia. *Early Childhood Research and Practice, 4*(1). http://ecrp.uiuc.edu/v4n1/ edwards.html.

Epstein, A. & Willhite, G. L. (2015). Teacher efficacy in an early childhood professional development school. *International Electronic Journal of Elementary Education, 7*(2), 189–198. https://iejee.com/index.php/IEJEE/article/view/7.

Gebbie, D., Ceglowski, D., Taylor, L., & Miels, J. (2011, March 1). The role of teacher efficacy in strengthening classroom support for preschool children with disabilities who exhibit challenging behaviors. https://www.researchgate.net/publication/257556840_The_Role_of_Teacher_Efficacy_in_Strengthening_Classroom_Support_for_Preschool_Children_with_Disabilities_Who_Exhibit_Challenging_Behaviors.

Guerra, A.L., Gidel, T., & Vezzetti, E. (2016). Toward a common procedure using Likert and Likert-type scales in small groups comparative design observations. International Design Conference: Dubrovnik, Croatia. https://www.researchgate.net/publication/307601241_Toward_a_common_procedure_using_likert_and_likert-type_scales_in_small_groups_comparative_design_observations.

Fuhs, M., Dale F., & Nesbitt, K. (2015). Prekindergarten children's executive functioning skills and achievement gains: The utility of direct assessments and teacher ratings. *Journal of Educational Psychology 107(1)*: 207– 21.

Kim, J. (2020). Learning and teaching online during COVID19: Experiences of student teachers in an early childhood education practicum. *International Journal of Early Childhood.*

Korkmaz, G. & Toraman, C. (2020). Are we ready for post COVID19 educational practice? An investigation into what educators think as to online learning. *International Journal of Technology in Education and Science.*

Leonhardt, M. (2020). 5 ways parents can help kids thrive amid remote learning. CNBC. https://www.cnbc.com/2020/10/01/5-ways-parents-can-help-kids-thrive-amid-remote-learning.html.

Leonhardt, M. (2020). Remote learning: Parents struggle with remote learning while working from home. CNBC. https://www.cnbc.com/2020/09/17/remote-learning-why-parents-feel-theyre-failing-with-back-to-school-from-home.html.

Mader, J. (2018). Does online preschool work. The Hechinger Report. https://www.pbs.org/newshour/education/online-programs-are-filling-a-preschool-gap-experts-warn-its-no- substitute-for-face-to-face-learning.

Norman, G. (2010). Likert scales, levels of measurement and the "laws" of statistics. *Advances in health sciences education: theory and practice, 15,* 625-32. doi: 10.1007/s10459-010-9222-y.

Pattnaik, J., & Jalongo, M. R. (2022). *The impact of covid-19 on Early Childhood Education and care: International Perspectives, challenges, and responses.* Springer.

Piaget, J. (1932). *The Moral Judgment of the Child.* London: Kegan Paul. London, United Kingdom.

Pinchevsky, N. & Bogler, R. (2018). The influence of teachers' perceived self-efficacy and role impact on their preferences in adopting strategies to resolve conflict situations with students. https://lej.cuchicago.edu/research-in-education/teacher-empowerment-and-teacher-perceptions-of-the- principals-servant-leadership/.

Plotka, R. & Guirguis, R. (2020). Training early childhood educators online: Lessons learned during the COVID-19 health crisis. *New York Academy of Public Education Professional Journal, 9,* 29-35.

Rimm-Kaufman, S., Pianta R., and Cox, M. (2000). Teachers' judgments of problems in the transition to kindergarten. *Early Childhood Research Quarterly, 15*(2): 147–66.

Singh, S., Roy, D., Sinha, K., Parveen, S., Sharma, G., & Joshi, G. (2020). Impact of COVID-19 and lockdown on mental health of children and adolescents: A narrative review with recommendations. *Psychiatry research,* 293, 113429. doi: 10.1016/j.psychres.2020.113429.

Skaalvik, E. & Skaalvik, S. (2010). Teacher self-efficacy and teacher burnout: A study of relations. *Teaching and Teacher Education, 26,* 1059–1069.

Stipek, D. (2012). Context matters: Effects of student characteristics and perceived administrative and parental support on teacher self-efficacy. *The Elementary School Journal, 112*(4), 590-606. doi:10.1086/664489.

Szente, J. (2020). Live virtual sessions with toddlers and preschoolers amid COVID19: implications for early childhood teacher education. *Journal of Technology and Teacher Education.*

Theodotou, E. & Kulovana, H. (2012). Virtual learning: examination of ICT as a beneficial learning tool for children's social development. Piraeus: Hellenic Educational Society.

Tschannen-Moran, M. & Hoy, A. W. (2001). Teacher efficacy: Capturing an elusive construct. *Teaching and Teacher Education, 17*(7), 783–805. doi: 10.1016/S0742-051X(01)00036-1.

Vygotsky, Lev S. (1978). *Mind in society: The development of higher psychological processes.* In M. Cole, John- Steiner, V. Scribner, S. and Souberman. E. (Eds.). Cambridge, MA: Harvard University Press.

Wahlstrom, K. & Louis, K. (2008). How teachers experience principal leadership: The roles of professional community, trust, efficacy, and shared responsibility. *Educational Administration Quarterly, 44*, 458–495.

Chapter 2
COVID-19, Virtual Learning, and Early Childhood Education Families' Experiences

The COVID-19 health crisis presented educators and families around the globe with the challenge of implementing remote learning for children. This challenge was especially pronounced for parents and educators of very young children (Szente, 2020). Early childhood education relies heavily on hands-on, play-based, collaborative learning experiences that are not easily implemented in online settings (Dodd-Nufrio, 2011). Furthermore, parents rely on early childhood education programs to support their children's social and emotional development; parents also rely on said programs for child care (Shrimali, 2020). Distance learning can be an effective way of meeting some early childhood goals but most likely not all. Little research has explored how distance learning has been effective at addressing family and educators' goals for early childhood education.

Virtual learning has been expanding in the United States and in the world even before the COVID-19 crisis. In the past decade, the number of students attending school online has grown significantly; in 2013, 31 states in the U.S. had schools that operated fully online (Currie-Rubin & Smith, 2014). Early childhood online instruction has also become more common. Programs such as the Upstart program have been providing online preschool instruction for thousands of children in the United States since 2013 (Mader, 2018). The program is funded by the United States federal government and provides online preschool education for young children in several U.S. states. As some degree of online instruction is expected to become more common in the future, the lessons learned during this pandemic might prove informative and even invaluable during this crisis and in future years. The lessons learned during the COVID-19 crisis might help inform future practices related to distance learning in early childhood.

Remote learning might have resulted in very different perceptions of children's experiences for teachers and families. In contrast to traditional in-person education, remote education has allowed families to observe and be involved in children's learning directly, while teachers rely on virtual observations (Buechner Institute for Governance, 2012). This way, remote learning has impacted the educators' ability to understand children's learning and social processes fully. At the same time, families had immediate exposure to their children's learning process. This shift has surely affected parents and teachers differently, and no studies have addressed these differences to date.

Furthermore, early childhood education is centered on strong partnerships between families and educators, as communication and support are central to children thriving (Buechner Institute for Governance, 2012). Little research has looked at family and educators' experiences with virtual communication during the COVID-19 health crisis. This study is unique as it takes into account the experiences of both families and teachers during the time of a universal health crisis of forced remote learning rather than optional online school enrollment.

Remote Learning in Early Childhood

Vygotsky's sociocultural theory asserts that young children learn through social interactions in their most immediate environment (Vygotsky, 1978). Vygotsky stressed the role of social activities in the educational process and the role of family and community as systems supporting child development and learning. The COVID-19 pandemic has shifted many of these interactions from the immediate environment to an online setting, modifying the roles of parents and educators.

The early childhood period is critical for establishing a trajectory for learning across one's lifespan (Montroy et al., 2016). Young children have specific social and emotional needs that require sustained adult interactions (Institute of Medicine and National Research Council, 2000). While the pandemic caused significant learning loss to children of all ages, young children suffered the most from distance learning because young children learn best with social interactions, hands-on exploration, sensory activities, music, and movement (Kuhfeld and Tarasawa, 2020).

Although educators around the world have struggled to adjust to providing online instruction, early childhood educators have faced unique challenges and have been the least prepared to provide online learning opportunities. For example, in the U.S., nearly all states have developed guidance and resources to support educators and families in remote learning during the pandemic, yet only a handful of states have developed remote learning models for early childhood. Most districts struggle with providing guidance and resources that are aligned with child development theories and practices (Donohue et al., 2021).

Furthermore, delivering effective early childhood education activities online requires an understanding of child development; this understanding is needed in order to develop a play-based sensorial learning experience that will keep young children engaged (Edwards, 2002). The developmental nature of young children requires the learning activities to be brief with a combination of visual and interactive activities, movement, music, games, and art (Hao, 2020). These activities have proven to be effective in the in-person context, yet little research has explored the effectiveness of these activities when implemented remotely; little research has taken into account the perspective of both parents and educators.

Despite the challenges of implementing remote learning activities with young children, educators have tried to implement several types of activities. Teachers have incorporated one-on-one activities, play-based learning, sing-alongs, book reading, and art activities (Edwards, 2002). Teachers also tried incorporating parents into the activities. Little research has explored what type of activities were considered most effective by educators during the pandemic when attempting to engage young children in remote learning. Similarly, little research has taken into account families' perceptions and experiences related to the effectiveness of such activities or the overlap between family and teacher perceptions.

Goals in Early Childhood Education for Families and Educators

Families and educators value several aspects of early childhood education. Families consider several goals and needs when enrolling their children in an early childhood education program. These goals and needs typically include preparing children for school, giving children the opportunity to socialize, and caregiving (Montroy et al., 2016). For example, a survey conducted by the United States National Center for Education Statistics of a nationally representative sample of parents of children enrolled in early childhood education programs found that 81% of parents reported that the learning activities were very important to them when choosing a program. These activities included learning the alphabet and numbers or other information that will prepare children for formal schooling (Mamedova et al., 2013). In addition, 71% of parents expected that early childhood programs would meet the need for their children to socialize and spend time with other children. Furthermore, 71% of parents indicated that caregiver availability and support were very important to them. Surprisingly, parents valued location and cost least as the location was only considered important to 59% of parents, and the cost was deemed important by 49% of parents (Mamedova et al., 2013).

While these goals play a key role in families' priorities for early childhood education, little research has explored whether parents felt that remote learning has been effective at meeting some or all of these needs. A survey conducted by the National Institute for Early Education Research (NIEER) has shown that 58% of parents were not satisfied with their children's remote preschool program (Barnett &

Jung, 2021). Yet, little research has explored which parental goals were met through remote education to a greater or lesser extent.

Family Needs and Challenges

In addition to providing children with a stimulating and supportive environment, both parents and educators understand that one big goal of early childhood education is providing child care. Two-thirds of children ages five and under have both parents employed in the labor force, meaning that children's early education programs are fundamental to parents' incomes. COVID-19 has changed the way families work and the care their children receive (Shrimali, 2020). Many parents have been juggling work with watching and educating children, often shift-splitting their schedules (if there are two parents at home), and waking up earlier or staying up later to get work done. Some have also moved in with their own parents, who are helping to watch their grandchildren (Greszler & Burke, 2020).

For online education to work, family engagement is critical. For children to be able to connect with their teachers and stay engaged in the lessons, an adult at home often has to take on this additional responsibility. During the crisis, parents often had to act as teachers and teacher aides. This is often a big task for the parents as they need to act as learning coaches while juggling other adult responsibilities (Barnett & Jung, 2021). They also need to take on roles for which they are untrained (Dong, 2020).

Research has shown that these stresses resulted in a decline in parental support for other home learning activities. Several parents reported a decline in reading books to their children. For example, in one study (Barnett & Jung, 2021), 85% of parents reported they read to their children three or more times per week before the pandemic started, yet only 71% of them read three times or more per week during the winter of 2021. Consequently, Read et al. (2021) suggest that families adapt to at-home learning by providing shared reading activities at home with young children. Specifically, reading became an activity the family maintained or replaced with other activities during the COVID-19 lockdown as they were able to maintain these positive routines along with providing the support and supervision children needed during shared reading activities. Yet, little research has explored the value parents placed on the child care aspects of early childhood education and how juggling multiple responsibilities might have affected families' experiences with distance learning.

Communication and Support

Partnership with families, support, and communication are central to early childhood education. Remote learning can prove challenging for communication between teachers and families (Leonhardt, 2020). However, virtual learning can also expand opportunities for communication and for the use of platforms that were not considered before the onset of the pandemic. In a study conducted in Norway, many families expressed that their communication with teachers increased during the pandemic. Parents shared that they were able to identify their children's struggles because they were exposed to their children's learning processes in their own homes. Parents felt they were more motivated to communicate with their children's teachers (Bubb & Jones, 2020). As a note, this study was conducted on elementary school-aged children. Early childhood education students were not part of that study as Bubb and Jones (2020) included students' survey responses which are more practical to collect from older students.

Communication with families is fundamental to early childhood practices, yet little is known about teachers' experiences with family communication in the virtual setting. In addition, little is known about the way teachers and families differ in their experiences of communicating and supporting during this period. This study aimed to explore perceptions of support from school administration, support from parents to teachers, support from teachers to parents, and increases in teacher-parent communication.

Research Questions

Online learning during the pandemic presented educators and families with unique opportunities and challenges. For the first time, parents had the opportunity to observe children learning firsthand, while teachers had to interact with children remotely; with this, remote learning might have resulted in very different perceptions of children's experiences for teachers and families.

Given the limited knowledge of families' and teachers' experiences during the pandemic, this study has attempted to address the gap in the literature by exploring the following research questions:

1. What goals in early childhood education are considered most important by educators and families?
2. How effectively did families and educators consider the online environment to be at achieving the main goals of early childhood education?
3. What specific activities were considered most effective at engaging children by educators and families?
4. To what extent did teachers and families experience communication and support?

Method

Participants

Participants were 53 preschool teachers teaching young children online due to the COVID-19 health crisis. In addition, 51 parents of young children learning online due to the COVID-19 health crisis participated in the study. The total sample was n = 104. This was part of a larger study exploring the effects of online education. All participants resided in a large metropolitan area in the U.S. Teachers and parents were not recruited from the same programs.

Table 2.1 describes the participants and shows the frequency and percentages of the type of early childhood education program in which the teachers taught and in which parents enrolled their children. The ages of the children in their classes ranged from 17 months old to 9 years of age, with a mean of 4.16 (*SD* = 1.52). The number of children in the classes ranged from 8 to 30, with a mean of 15.04 children (*SD* = 4.32). Parents described the age of the children as ranging from 2 to 8 years of age, with a mean of 4.69 (*SD* = 1.49).

Survey Item	*n*	%
School Description for Teachers:		
Public School	5	10.2
Private Preschool	9	18.4
Private Faith-Based/Parochial	6	12.2
Head Start	3	6.1
Universal Pre-Kindergarten	8	16.3
Child Care Program	15	30.6
Other publicly funded preschool program	3	6.1
Total	49*	100.0
School Description for Families:		
Public School	7	13.7
Private Preschool	10	19.6
Private Faith-Based/Parochial	18	35.3
Head Start	0	0.0
Universal Pre-Kindergarten	8	15.7
Child Care Program	5	9.8
Other publicly funded preschool program	3	5.9
Total	51	100.0

**Note*: Four teachers did not answer this question.

Table 2.1 *Participants: Frequency and Percentages*

Procedure and Instrument

Teachers and parents were asked to fill out an online survey about their experiences with young children learning online during the COVID-19 crisis. Only educators teaching young children solely online were recruited to fill out the survey. Teachers were recruited by word of mouth. Similarly, parents whose children were solely learning online were recruited for the study. Families were recruited by word of mouth and by several of the teachers who participated in the study.

To answer the research questions, a survey was developed in order to measure teacher and family experiences. Before the survey was administered, it was shared with small focus groups of preschool educators teaching online and with parents of young children learning online to ensure that it reflected common experiences. The survey was edited based on teachers' and parents' feedback. Item descriptions for the survey are provided in the results section in Table 2.2.

The survey was developed to assess the following constructs:

- Goals for Early Childhood Education: The survey asked teachers and parents to rate the importance of eight goals that are considered central to early childhood education. Respondents were asked to rate importance on a scale ranging from 1 (not important) to 4 (very important). Table 2.2 includes all the items.
- Effectiveness of the Online Environment in Meeting Early Childhood Education Goals: the survey asked teachers and parents to rate how effective online learning was with regard to addressing eight goals for early childhood education. Respondents were asked to rate the effectiveness on a scale ranging from 1 (not effective) to 4 (very effective).
- Effectiveness of Specific Activities: Teachers tried different online activities to engage young children during this time;

respondents were asked to rate the activities' effectiveness on a scale ranging from 1 (not effective) to 4 (very effective).

- Level of Communication and Support: Parents and teachers were asked to rate the four statements about communication and support from the school administration. Participants rated statements on a scale ranging from 1 (do not agree) to 4 (strongly agree).

Results

Descriptive Statistics

The descriptive statistics for the full sample are presented in Table 2.2. The survey items are presented in the order in which they were asked.

Survey item	Min	Max	*M*	*SD*
Activities that are most effective online				
Story time/reading books	1.00	4.00	2.89	.95
Games and social activities	1.00	4.00	2.93	.93
Direct Instruction	1.00	4.00	2.47	.88
Sing-alongs	1.00	4.00	2.74	.98
One-on-one time with teachers	1.00	4.00	3.12	.87
Hands-on activities with an adult assisting	1.00	4.00	3.00	.90
Hands-on activities without adult assisting	1.00	4.00	2.00	.88
Art activities	1.00	4.00	2.71	.94
Goals in Early Childhood Education				
Supporting family child care needs	1.00	4.00	3.61	.77
Helping children learn the alphabet, the numbers, or other information that will prepare them for school	1.00	4.00	3.38	.81
Helping children make friends	1.00	4.00	3.66	.61
Helping children interact with other children positively	3.00	4.00	3.85	.35
Giving children the opportunity to play	2.00	4.00	3.80	.44

Survey item	Min	Max	*M*	*SD*
Helping children learn how to follow rules	2.00	4.00	3.58	.58
Helping children learn about appropriate behaviors	2.00	4.00	3.76	.44
Helping children learn about classrooms routines and schedules	2.00	4.00	3.58	.61
Effectiveness of the online environment at supporting EC goals				
Supporting child care needs	1.00	4.00	2.27	1.12
Helping children learn the alphabet, the numbers, or other information that will prepare them for school	1.00	4.00	2.52	.91
Helping children make friends	1.00	4.00	1.81	1.00
Helping children interact with other children positively	1.00	4.00	2.17	1.01
Giving children the opportunity to play	1.00	4.00	2.12	1.10
Helping children learn how to follow rules	1.00	4.00	2.23	.96
Helping children learn about appropriate behaviors	1.00	4.00	2.25	.92
Helping children learn about classrooms routines and schedules so they are prepared for school	1.00	4.00	2.14	1.03
Communication and Support				
I felt supported by school administration	1.00	4.00	3.24	.70
I felt supported by the families/teachers in the program	1.00	4.00	3.18	.71
I was able to keep open communication with families/teachers	1.00	4.00	3.37	.61
Communication with families/teachers actually increased or became more open	1.00	4.00	3.28	.72

Table 2.2 *Descriptive Statistics for the Survey Questions (n = 104)*

Research Question 1: What goals in early childhood education are considered most important to educators and families?

The survey asked teachers and parents to rate the importance of eight early childhood education goals. The descriptive statistics presented in Table 2.2 show that the sample prioritized social goals over academic goals. Participants scored "helping children interact with other children positively," as most important, followed by "giving children the opportunity to play" and "helping children learn about appropriate behaviors." The participants found "helping children learn the alphabet, the numbers, or other information that will prepare them for school" as the least important for early childhood education.

Do teachers and families differ in their goals for early childhood education?

A one-way ANOVA was used to determine if there were statistically significant differences in the average perceived effectiveness of online learning for helping children learn the alphabet, the numbers, or other information that will prepare them for school (teachers vs family). An ANOVA is an extension of the independent samples t-test which can be used to compare any number of groups or treatments (Bewick et al., 2004) and to control for Type I error (Kao et al., 2008). Levene's test of equality of error variances was not statistically significant ($F(1,102) = 0.32$, $p = .56$), indicating this assumption of normality was not violated.

The descriptive statistics by respondent type and the ANOVAs appear in Table 2.3. The results show that families and educators were consistent in the goals for early childhood education, and their answers did not differ significantly. Yet, Table 2.3 indicated that there was a statistically significant difference in the average perceived importance of "supporting family child care needs" by type of respondent, as it was rated as more important for teachers than for families.

Variable	Teacher			Family			ANOVA				
Survey Question	N	M	SD	N	M	SD	Effect	*df*	*F*	*p*	η^2
Supporting family needs*	53	3.84	0.36	51	3.37	0.99	Between Groups	1	10.61	.002*	.094
							Within Groups	102			
							Total	103			
Helping children learn the alphabet, the numbers, or other information that will prepare them for school	53	3.32	0.80	51	3.45	0.83	Between Groups	1	0.65	.41	.006
							Within Groups	102			
							Total	103			
Helping children make friends	53	3.64	0.62	51	3.68	0.61	Between Groups	1	0.13	.71	.001
							Within Groups	102			
							Total	103			
Helping children interact with other children positively	53	3.84	0.36	51	3.86	0.34	Between Groups	1	0.03	.84	.000
							Within Groups	102			
							Total	103			

Variable	Teacher			Family			ANOVA				
Survey Question	N	M	SD	N	M	SD	Effect	*df*	*F*	*p*	η^2
Giving children the opportunity to play	53	3.78	0.45	51	3.82	0.43	Between Groups	1	0.15	.69	.002
							Within Groups	101			
							Total	102			
Helping children learn how to follow rules	53	3.52	0.57	51	3.64	0.59	Between Groups	1	1.07	.30	.010
							Within Groups	102			
							Total	103			
Helping children learn about appropriate behaviors	53	3.71	0.49	51	3.82	0.38	Between Groups	1	1.49	.22	.014
							Within Groups	102			
							Total	103			
Helping children learn about classrooms routines and schedules	53	3.58	0.60	51	3.58	0.63	Between Groups	1	0.001	.97	.000
							Within Groups	102			
							Total	103			

Table 2.3 *Descriptive Statistics and ANOVA Results for Importance of Goals by Type of Respondent*

Research Question 2: How effectively did families and educators consider the online environment to be at achieving the main goals of early childhood education?

The descriptive statistics presented in Table 2.4 show that the sample did not consider the online environment particularly effective at meeting its goals. When asked to score the importance of each goal (Table 2.3), most goals received high scores ranging between 3.38 and 3.80, indicating "important" to "very important." Yet, when asked to score the effectiveness of the online environment in meeting those goals (Table 2.4), scores ranged from 1.81 to 2.52, indicating that participants considered the online environment somewhere between "not effective" and "somewhat effective." Despite the participants rating social skills as the most important goals and academic skills as least important, participants rated the online environment as most effective at fostering academic skills and least effective at promoting friendships and social skills.

Do families and educators differ in their perception of online education effectiveness?

The results show several differences in the way families and educators experienced the effectiveness of online education in achieving their goals for early childhood education. In general, educators had a more optimistic view, while families had more negative experiences. For example, results in Table 2.4 indicate that there was a statistically significant difference in the average perceived effectiveness of online learning for supporting family child care needs by type of respondent. In addition, there was a statistically significant difference in the average perceived effectiveness of online learning for helping children make friends, helping children interact with other children positively, giving children the opportunity to play, and helping children learn about appropriate behaviors. As seen in Table 2.4, teachers perceived statistically significant higher levels of effectiveness of online learning for all those goals.

Furthermore, Table 2.4 indicates there was a trend toward statistical significance in the difference in average perceived effectiveness of online learning for helping children learn the alphabet, the numbers, or other information that will prepare them for school by type of respondent. Similarly, there was a marginally significant difference in the average perceived effectiveness of online learning in helping children learn how to follow the rules. The average perceived effectiveness was marginally higher for teachers than for families. Lastly, there was no statistically significant difference in the average perceived effectiveness of online learning for helping children learn about classroom routines and schedules by type of respondent.

Variable	Teachers			Family			ANOVA				
Survey Question	N	M	SD	N	M	SD	Effect	*df*	*F*	*p*	η^2
Supporting family need	53	2.94	0.86	51	1.58	0.94	Between Groups	1	58.52	.001*	.365
							Within Groups	102			
							Total	103			
Helping children learn the alphabet, the numbers, or other information that will prepare them for school	53	2.67	0.93	51	0.94	0.87	Between Groups	1	2.98	.08	.028
							Within Groups	102			
							Total	103			
Helping children make friends	53	2.01	0.99	51	1.60	0.98	Between Groups	1	4.51	.03*	.042
							Within Groups	102			
							Total	103			

Variable	Teachers			Family			ANOVA				
Survey Question	N	M	SD	N	M	SD	Effect	*df*	*F*	*p*	η^2
Helping children interact with other children positively	53	2.54	0.95	51	1.78	0.94	Between Groups	1	16.81	.001*	.142
							Within Groups	102			
							Total	103			
Giving children the opportunity to play	53	2.54	1.06	51	1.68	0.96	Between Groups	1	18.51	.001*	.154
							Within Groups	102			
							Total	103			
Helping children learn how to follow rules	53	2.39	0.96	51	2.05	0.94	Between Groups	1	3.22	.07	.031
							Within Groups	102			
							Total	103			

Variable	Teachers			Family				ANOVA			
Survey Question	N	M	SD	N	M	SD	Effect	*df*	*F*	*p*	η^2
Helping children learn about appropriate behaviors	53	2.43	0.88	51	2.07	0.93	Between Groups	1	3.95	.04*	.037
							Within Groups	102			
							Total	103			
Helping children learn about classrooms routines and schedules so they are prepared for school	53	2.13	1.05	51	2.156	1.02	Between Groups	1	.01	.90	.001
							Within Groups	102			
							Total	103			

Table 2.4 *Descriptive Statistics and ANOVA Results for the Effectiveness of Online Learning for Addressing Eight Goals*

Research Question 3: What specific activities did educators and families consider most effective at engaging children?

Teachers have tried to implement several types of developmentally appropriate activities in order to engage children during this time. When looking at specific activities, the attention of an adult made a big difference. For example, the most effective activity type was one-on-one time with a teacher. Similarly, the sample rated hands-on activities with an adult assisting as effective (M = 3.00) and hands-on activities without an adult assisting as somewhat effective (M = 2.00). The sample considered games social activities and storytime as more effective than direct instruction, sing-alongs, or art.

Did educators and families differ in their perceptions of the effectiveness of specific activities?

The results presented in Table 2.5 show that families and teachers rated the effectiveness of specific activities similarly. Teachers were slightly more optimistic than families when rating the effectiveness of specific activities. For example, there was a marginally statistically significant difference in the scores of average effectiveness of storytime/reading books by type of respondent, and educators scored this activity as more effective than families. In addition, as seen in Table 2.5, there was a statistically significant difference in the average effectiveness of sing-alongs by type of respondent, and the average perceived effectiveness rating of sing-alongs was higher for teachers in comparison to families.

Variable	Teachers			Family			ANOVA				
Survey Question	N	M	SD	N	M	SD	Effect	*df*	*F*	*p*	η^2
Story time/ reading books	53	3.05	0.86	51	2.72	1.02	Between Groups	1	3.19	.07	.030
							Within Groups	102			
							Total	103			
Games and social activities	53	3.07	0.89	51	2.78	0.96	Between Groups	1	2.54	.11	.024
							Within Groups	102			
							Total	103			
Direct Instruction	53	2.39	0.81	51	2.54	0.94	Between Groups	1	.78	.37	.008
							Within Groups	102			
							Total	103			

Variable	Teachers			Family			ANOVA				
Survey Question	N	M	SD	N	M	SD	Effect	*df*	*F*	*p*	η^2
Sing-alongs*	53	3.05	0.79	51	2.41	1.06	Between Groups	1	12.36	.001*	.108
							Within Groups	102			
							Total	103			
One-on-one time with teachers	53	3.13	0.83	51	3.11	0.93	Between Groups	1	.007	.93	.001
							Within Groups	102			
							Total	103			
Hands-on activities with an adult assisting	53	2.94	0.94	51	3.07	0.86	Between Groups	1	.57	.45	.006
							Within Groups	102			
							Total	103			

Variable	Teachers			Family			ANOVA				
Survey Question	N	M	SD	N	M	SD	Effect	*df*	*F*	*p*	η^2
Hands-on activities without adult assisting	53	1.96	0.80	51	2.03	0.95	Between Groups	1	.19	.65	.002
							Within Groups	102			
							Total	103			
Art activities	53	2.77	0.93	51	2.64	0.95	Between Groups	1	.46	.49	.005
							Within Groups	102			
							Total	103			

Table 2.5 *Descriptive Statistics and ANOVA Results for Average Effectiveness Ratings by Type of Respondent*

Research Question 4: To what extent did teachers and families experience communication and support?

The descriptive statistics presented in Table 2.6 show that both families and educators felt a great deal of support from their respective school administrations; they felt they were able to maintain effective communication between families and teachers, and many felt that communication increased while children were learning online. This was reflected in their high scores for all four items in the survey.

Did families and teachers differ in their experiences of communication and support?

An ANOVA was used to determine if there were statistically significant differences in average perceived support and types of communication during online teaching and learning. Table 2.6 shows the descriptive statistics for average perceived support and communication during online learning by type of respondent. As seen in Table 2.6, there was a statistically significant difference in the average support felt by teachers and families during online learning by type of respondent, $F(1,102) = 7.68$, $p = .007$. Specifically, families reported feeling marginally more supported by their respective school administrators than teachers did. Families experienced significantly more support from teachers than teachers felt supported by families.

Variable	Teachers			Family			ANOVA				
	N	M	SD	N	M	SD	Effect	*df*	*F*	*p*	η^2
I felt supported by administration	53	3.11	0.80	51	3.37	0.56	Between Groups	1	3.62	.06	.034
							Within Groups	102			
							Total	103			
I felt supported by teachers/families	53	3.0	0.78	51	3.37	.56	Between Groups	1	7.68	.007	.070
							Within Groups	102			
							Total	103			
Open communication	53	3.33	.65	51	3.39	.57	Between Groups	1	.192	.66	.002
							Within Groups	102			
							Total	103			
Increased communication	53	3.21	.79	51	3.35	.63	Between Groups	1	1.07	.30	.010
							Within Groups	102			
							Total	103			

Table 2.6 *Descriptive Statistics and ANOVA Results for Administrative Support and Communication by Type of Respondent*

Discussion

The COVID-19 health crisis has presented early childhood educators and families with unique challenges. At the same time, it has provided the opportunity to explore online learning in early childhood. The roles of teachers and families have shifted during this time, forcing teachers to interact with young children through a screen. In contrast, families had the opportunity to observe and facilitate learning in person while fulfilling other obligations such as work. This situation has resulted in educators and families navigating the learning process differently. This study has attempted to explore and compare the experiences of families and educators during this challenging time. This study is unique as it has taken into account the perspectives of both families and teachers.

The present study explored four questions. First, the study assessed the goals in early childhood education that were considered most important by educators and families. Second, this study explored how effective families and educators consider the online environment in achieving the main goals of early childhood education. Third, the study explored what specific activities educators and parents considered most effective in engaging children. Lastly, the study assessed to what extent teachers and families experienced communication and support.

Parents' and Teachers' Goals in Early Childhood Education (ECE)

The first research question explored parents' and teachers' goals in early childhood education and found that parents and teachers were consistent in their goals and objectives. Specifically, parents and teachers valued opportunities for socialization and play most. During this tumultuous period, both parents and teachers felt that school readiness was the least prioritized goal for their children. Research conducted before the pandemic has shown that parents value learning activities as much or more than socialization opportunities (Mamedova et al., 2013). The lack of socialization opportunities in the online environment might have played a role in heightening the value of socialization and play during this time.

Effectiveness of the Online Environment and ECE Goals

The second research question explored the effectiveness of the online environment in meeting early childhood education goals. Both parents and teachers found that the online environment was not very effective at meeting their goals. Despite the rating of socialization and play as the most important in early childhood education, they found that this goal was least likely to be accomplished effectively through virtual learning. Similarly, the online environment was rated most effective at fostering academic skills, even though this was the goal least valued by both parents and teachers. Nevertheless, teachers were significantly more optimistic than parents when evaluating the effectiveness of online education in accomplishing early childhood education goals. Educators rated virtual education as significantly more effective than parents did when it came to supporting child care needs, helping children make friends, helping children interact with other children positively, giving children the opportunity to play, and helping children learn about appropriate behaviors. Similarly, educators rated online learning as marginally more effective than parents when it came to helping children learn how to follow the rules and learn academic skills. Hu et al. (2021) emphasized the importance of family engagement and support as two aspects that influence young learners' online learning experiences.

Families and Teachers: Children's Engagement

The third research question explored the way families and teachers experienced children's engagement and participation. Teachers tried a variety of developmentally appropriate activities to engage young children in learning. Teachers and parents rated children's engagement similarly, and both agreed that the availability of adult attention made a big difference in children's participation and learning. For example, the most effective activity type was one-on-one time with a teacher. Similarly, families and teachers rated hands-on activities with an adult assisting as more effective than when an adult was not assisting.

Nevertheless, families had more negative perspectives than educators when judging the effectiveness of specific online activities, and they rated story time and sing-alongs as less effective than educators did. The reasons for more negative perceptions in parents than in teachers might be because families saw their children first-hand and perceived them as less engaged and more distracted during these activities than educators were able to see. In addition, during the pandemic, families increased their reading of books and other in-person activities with their children, and this might have led them to perceive online activities as less effective.

Families and Teachers: Support and Communication

Lastly, the fourth research question explored the level of support and communication that teachers and families experienced during this time. The results have shown that both groups experienced a great deal of support from the school administration; they felt they were able to maintain effective communication, and many felt that communication increased while children were learning online. Nevertheless, families felt more support than teachers did from respective school administrations. Similarly, families felt more supported by teachers than teachers felt by families.

Limitations

This study has several limitations. First, this research relies solely on survey data because of the pandemic. Observational tools will further enrich the study of family and educators' experiences while attempting to engage young children with online learning.

Second, the study consisted of a small sample in a large metropolitan area in the U.S. The pandemic presented a unique opportunity to study a worldwide phenomenon. Shaik (2022) explored the challenges early childhood providers face in South Africa - specifically, the changes made to address the technological inequities in economically disadvantaged communities. Nonetheless, further research is necessary to explore these processes in international contexts and varied settings such as rural or suburban neighborhoods.

Lastly, this study explored the experiences of children who were solely learning online. Further research is necessary to establish the effectiveness of combined methods in early childhood. Past research has shown that pre-service teachers training to become early childhood educators did not consider taking classes solely online effective. Yet, they valued a combination of in-person and online instruction (Plotka & Guirguis, 2020). Further research can explore the effectiveness of the combination of online and in-person experiences for young children. It is possible that when given the opportunity to socialize in person on some days, young children will benefit from storytime or other online interactions with children and teachers they often see.

Lessons Learned and Implications for the Future

As online early childhood education is expected to expand around the world, the lessons learned during the pandemic should prove informative for working with young children and their families, specifically the lessons learned regarding families and educators' values of early childhood education, both groups' online experience, and the level of communication and support experienced by both groups.

One of the most important lessons learned was that families and educators were aligned in their values for their children's education and their experiences with online learning. Yet, they did not find the online classroom was highly effective in meeting their children's goals. Their most important goals of socialization and play had suffered the most within the online environment. Socialization and play are cornerstones of early childhood education, and expanding online learning might result in a delay in the development of these fundamental skills. The results of the present study have shown that online environments are more effective at facilitating academic skills. By shifting early childhood programs online, school readiness might be prioritized at the expense of socio-emotional development and well-being.

Another important lesson learned was that, in general, families had more negative experiences than educators, while educators were more optimistic about online learning. Virtual teaching makes it harder for educators to "read" children's experiences, making it easy to overestimate their ability to engage children in learning activities. At the same time, with direct contact with children, families were able to perceive more gaps in children's experiences.

Overall, online learning can generate a mismatch between families' and educators' experiences and can lead educators to misunderstand children's experiences. Furthermore, both families and teachers agreed that for activities to be effective an adult at home needs to spend a substantial amount of time guiding children. This can take a toll on parents who are juggling work and other responsibilities, leading parents to rate online learning more negatively. Further research can explore whether families with fewer responsibilities, such as those who are not working from home or who do not have multiple caregiving responsibilities, have more positive attitudes towards remote learning. Similarly, since these conditions are tightly related to socioeconomic status, further research can explore whether families with more resources experience virtual learning more positively.

Finally, the last important lesson was that virtual learning is an adequate environment for supporting parent-teacher communication. This should be considered for future practice as education programs can expand the modes of communication with parents and facilitate family-school connections through virtual platforms not used before the pandemic. The findings of this study and the lessons learned during the COVID-19 pandemic should prove useful in future years as parents and educators navigate new ways to learn, teach, work, and communicate.

References

Barnett, W. S., & Jung, K. (2021). *Seven impacts of the pandemic on young children and their parents: Initial findings from NIEER's December 2020 preschool learning activities Survey.* National Institute for Early Education Research. https://nieer.org/wp-content/uploads/2021/02/NIEER_Seven_Impacts_of_the_Pandemic_on_Young_Children_and_their_Parents.pdf

Bewick, V., Cheek, L., & Ball, J. (2004). Statistics review 9: One-way analysis of variance. *Critical Care, 8*(2), 130–136. https://doi.org/10.1186/cc2836

Bubb, S., & Jones, M.-A. (2020). Learning from the COVID-19 home-schooling experience: Listening to pupils, parents/caregivers and teachers. *Improving Schools, 23*(3), 209–222. https://doi.org/10.1177/1365480220958797

Buechner Institute for Governance. (2012). *A study of online learning: Perspectives of online learners and educators*. https://www.cde.state.co.us/sites/default/files/documents/onlinelearning/download/study

Currie-Rubin, R., & Smith, S. J. (2014). Understanding the roles of families in virtual learning. *TEACHING Exceptional Children, 46*(5), 117–126. https://doi.org/10.1177/0040059914530101

Dodd-Nufrio, A. T. (2011). Reggio Emilia, Maria Montessori, and John Dewey: Dispelling teachers' misconceptions and understanding theoretical foundations. *Early Childhood Education Journal, 39*(4), 235–237. https://doi.org/10.1007/s10643-011-0451-3

Donohue, C., Johnson, A., Lucas, P., Lynd, C., Mukerjee, J., & Thouvenelle, S. (2021). *Distance learning and early childhood education*. Head Start ECLKC. https://eclkc.ohs.acf.hhs.gov/archive/professional-development/article/distance-learning-early-childhood-education

Dong, C., Cao, S., & Li, H. (2020). Young Children's online learning during COVID-19 pandemic: Chinese parents' beliefs and attitudes. *Children and Youth Services Review, 118*, 105440. https://doi.org/10.1016/j.childyouth.2020.105440

Edwards, C. P. (2002). Three Approaches from Europe: Waldorf, Montessori, and Reggio Emilia. *Faculty Publications, Department of Child, Youth, and Family Studies, 4*(1), 1–24. https://digitalcommons.unl.edu/cgi/viewcontent.cgi?article=1001&context=famconfacpub

Greszler, R., & Burke, L. (2020). *Rethinking early childhood education and child care in the COVID-19 era*. The Heritage Foundation. https://www.heritage.org/education/report/rethinking-early-childhood-education-and-child care-the-covid-19-era

Hao, W. (2020). *Remote learning in early childhood. policy update*. National Association of State Boards of Education. https://eric.ed.gov/?id=ED609777 Institute of Medicine and National Research Council. (2000). *From neurons to neighborhoods: The science of early childhood development*. The National Academies Press. https://doi.org/10.17226/9824

Kao, L. S., & Green, C. E. (2008). Analysis of variance: Is there a difference in means and what does it mean? *Journal of Surgical Research, 144*(1), 158–170. https://doi.org/10.1016/j.jss.2007.02.053

Kuhfeld, M., & Tarasawa, B. (2020). *The COVID-19 slide: What summer learning loss can tell us about the potential impact of school closures on student academic achievement*. NWEA. https://www.nwea.org/research/publication/the-covid-19-slide-what-summer-learning-loss

Leonhardt, M. (2020, September 17). *Parents struggle with remote learning while working from home: "I'm constantly failing."* CNBC. Retrieved July 12, 2022, from https://www.cnbc.com/2020/09/17/remote-learning-why-parents-feel-theyre-failing-with-back-to-school-from-home.html

Mader, J. (2020, October 21). *Experts call for an end to online preschool programs*. The Hechinger Report. https://hechingerreport.org/experts-call-for-an-end-to-online-preschool-programs/

Mamedova, S., Zuckerberg, A., & Redford, J. (2019). *Early childhood program participation, from the national household education surveys program of 2012*. National Center for Education Statistics (NCES). https://nces.ed.gov/pubs2013/2013029rev2.pdf

Montroy, J. J., Bowles, R. P., Skibbe, L. E., McClelland, M. M., & Morrison, F. J. (2016). The development of self-regulation across early childhood. *Developmental Psychology, 52*(11), 1744–1762. https://doi.org/10.1037/dev0000159

Plotka, R., & Guirguis, R. (2020). Lessons learned during the COVID-19 health crisis. *The New York Academy of Public Education Research Journal, 9*(1), 29–35. https://doi.org/https://nyape.org/wp-content/uploads/2020/12/NYAPE-research-journal-2020.pdf

Read, K., Gaffney, G., Chen, A., & Imran, A. (2021). The impact of COVID-19 on families' home literacy practices with young children. *Early Childhood Education Journal*. https://doi.org/10.1007/s10643-021-01270-6

Shaik, N. (2022). Transforming teaching and learning in early childhood care and education during COVID-19 in a poor community of the Cape Flats, South Africa. *Early Childhood Education Journal*. https://doi.org/10.1007/s10643-022-01329-y

Shrimali, B. P. (2020). *Child Care, COVID-19, and our Economic Future*. Federal Reserve Bank of San Francisco. https://www.frbsf.org/community-development/publications/community

Szente, J. (2020). Live virtual sessions with toddlers and preschoolers amid COVID-19: Implications for early childhood teacher education. *Journal of Technology and Teacher Education, 28*(2), 373-380. https://www.learntechlib.org/primary/p/216174/

Vygotsky, L. S. (1978). *Mind in Society: The Development of Higher Psychological Processes*. Cambridge, MA: Harvard University Press.

Chapter 3

Higher Education and the Perspectives of Teacher Preparation Programs in Early Childhood Education

Early childhood teacher preparation programs train teacher candidates to engage young children in hands-on, multisensory, and multidisciplinary social learning experiences while involving families and communities. In recent years, higher education programs have shifted towards online instruction (Govindarajan & Srivastava, 2020). However, it is unclear whether the online environment is an effective platform for training teachers in supporting young children's development and learning. Similarly, while the assumption is that many young adults prefer online learning, it is uncertain whether this preference extends to young adults training to become teachers of young children. This study attempts to explore teacher candidate experiences and preferences related to remote learning while training to become early childhood educators.

The novel COVID-19 health crisis has forced early childhood teacher education programs in many parts of the world to shift teacher preparation to the online setting. This situation has presented the opportunity to explore the effectiveness of online training for early childhood teacher candidates. Higher education institutions have been shifting coursework to remote learning in the past years, and this shift is expected to continue to grow, even after the health crisis has been overcome (Govindarajan & Srivastava, 2020). This study proposes that the opinions of teacher candidates should help inform this shift.

Theoretical Background

The assumptions that learning is an active process fostered by an environment that supports exploration, manipulation, social interactions, and play are at the core of the early childhood education field. These assumptions are based on the works of theorists such as Piaget and Vygotsky as well as the main early childhood educational approaches such as Reggio Emilia and Montessori (Dodd-Nufrio, 2011; Edwards, 2002).

Piaget (1972) believed that children are active learners and create knowledge by manipulating the environment around them. Piaget considered that children act as "little scientists" developing hypotheses and testing them throughout play and exploration, and therefore inadvertently learning through their conclusions. From an early age, children conduct research on the world around them through their senses, by coordinating experiences from physical and motor interactions with objects. Children progress from manipulating objects to developing the ability to manipulate symbols. Symbolic play is one of the main ways children use symbols and ideas to explore and understand the world. Similarly, the use of language, drawing, and eventually writing, constitute symbols that give children the ability to explore, categorize, organize, and understand ideas about the world around them. Thus, according to Piaget, learning is based on active exploration of the physical world.

Like Piaget, Vygotsky (1978) believed that young children make meaning of their world through learning environments that support social interactions. Young children develop emotion, language, meaning, and knowledge with the help of peers, older children, and adults. Stimulating and supportive social interactions within the family and community provide the ideal setting for learning. Thus, according to Vygotsky, learning is a social process.

Most contemporary approaches to early childhood education incorporate these theoretical backgrounds and stress the need for curriculum and educational environments that support active learning, exploration, play, and socialization. For example, the Reggio Emilia approach to early childhood education prioritizes exploration through play, music, and the arts (Dodd-Nufrio, 2011). Similarly, the Montessori approach stresses hands-on learning and exploration of materials and manipulatives (Edwards, 2002).

The theories and approaches to early childhood education that stress hands-on exploration and socialization tend to be at odds with remote learning and the virtual environment, making early childhood teacher candidates less likely to appreciate this mode of instruction. This study aims to explore this assumption.

Key Competencies for Early Childhood Teacher Preparation Programs

The National Association for the Education of Young Children (NAEYC, 2019) outlines key competencies for effective teachers in early childhood education. These competencies are integrated into early childhood education teacher preparation programs throughout the United States and guide the framework, objectives, coursework, and outcomes for programs.

NAEYC (2019) proposes that early childhood educators must integrate knowledge from all aspects of a child's development. This encompasses several disciplines including family dynamics, mental health, speech and language therapy, special education, and bilingual education. Early childhood teachers must integrate multiple sources of knowledge into a coherent approach in order to support young children's development and guide/support their respective families. With this, becoming an early childhood educator is a complex process and requires candidates to be competent in many disciplines, in addition to classroom instruction and management.

A key competency for teachers is to understand current research in child development, including cognitive, language, social, emotional, and physical development, and the extent to which these areas in development are interrelated. Educators must be trained to consider the critical role of relationships and interactions, and the role of play in development (NAEYC, 2019). In addition, educators must recognize the role of adverse early life experiences, including the role of inequality, socioeconomic class and immigration, and other factors that affect development. Furthermore, teachers must be familiar with the identification of delays or disabilities and the use of individualized supports needed to help children reach their potential (NAEYC, 2019). Effective programs prepare teachers who collaborate with families by providing training on effective communication skills that respect linguistic and cultural diversity. They connect families with community resources in order to better support the development of young children (NAEYC, 2019).

In addition, a fundamental competency for teacher candidates is to learn to craft a developmentally appropriate curriculum that engages young children in exploration. Teachers need to be prepared to employ a diverse array of practices in order to deliver curriculum strategies in effective ways and engage young children in stimulating and challenging learning experiences (NAEYC, 2019). Educators must acquire the ability to support language development, foster literacy skills, engage young children in scientific inquiry, as well as interest them in learning about social studies and the community around them. Effective programs prepare candidates to use multiple observation and assessment strategies in order to fully understand a child's development and progress in learning in order to tailor instruction for children's individual needs (NAEYC, 2019).

Lastly, a key competency in teachers of young children is the ability to create a positive and safe environment in which children learn about appropriate social behaviors in developmentally appropriate ways. This involves supporting the emotional needs of every child and creating opportunities for socialization and positive social development through healthy peer interactions (NAEYC, 2019).

These key competencies of early childhood education elucidate the collaborative, interdisciplinary, hands-on nature of the early childhood education field. These competencies require teacher education programs to employ a variety of instructional strategies that do not always translate well to the virtual environment. This study aims to explore how these competencies are met in the virtual environment.

Teachers' Priorities and Goals in Early Childhood Education

As discussed, early childhood teacher education programs train individuals to collaborate with families in meaningful ways and to team up with other professionals with an interdisciplinary approach to support children's growth in all areas of development, including motor development and speech. Because of their training and their choice of profession, it is possible to assume that most early childhood professionals tend to value teamwork, group work, and learning through social interactions in in-person environments. For higher education students choosing this career, social networking and building a community of educators might be an important goal in their educational experience, in addition to learning content and being granted a degree. For this reason, it is possible to assume that teacher candidates in early childhood will prioritize in-person education more than students in other fields. However, little research addresses this question.

In addition, educators tend to view the most important goals of early childhood education differently from one another. Educators of young children prioritize different areas of development depending on the early childhood program philosophy, approach, and major goals. For example, programs like High Scope or Head Start have as one of the most important goals to develop academic skills in young children in order to better prepare them for school (High Scope, 2020). The Reggio

Emilia approach to early childhood education results in preschool classrooms that value self-expression, art, and community exploration (Dodd-Nufrio, 2011). Montessori schools prioritize self-regulation skills in young children, while many programs have socialization, play, and the development of friendships as the main goal of their curriculum (Edwards, 2002).

For this reason, teachers and teacher candidates view their roles and the most important goals in early childhood education differently from one another. Some view play and exploration as the most important goal in early childhood education and facilitate this process as the teacher's main role. Some teachers value socialization opportunities, while others prioritize academic knowledge and school readiness. Some of the skills to support teachers' priorities and goals are harder to develop in a remote learning environment than others. For example, training teachers to deliver content knowledge might be easier to do online than training teachers to help children regulate their emotions or behaviors. Because different teacher candidates might have different goals in the education of young children and might see their role as a teacher differently, they will also experience remote learning differently. Yet, very little research was conducted to answer these questions.

Gap in the Literature and Research Questions

Higher education has increasingly shifted to online instruction. The assumption is that young adults prefer virtual learning (Lederman, 2019). Yet, little is known about the preferences of early childhood teacher candidates. At the same time, the early childhood teacher preparation field guidelines demand training teachers in the use of a multidisciplinary, collaborative team approach while fostering child learning through interactions, exploration, and play (NAEYC, 2019). Very little is known about how effectively these skills can be learned through online instruction. Similarly, early childhood preparation programs attempt to foster key competencies in new teachers and some of these competencies might be easier to achieve in a virtual format than others.

In addition, contemporary early childhood education approaches such as those Reggio Emilia, Montessori, Head Start or High Scope differ significantly in their goal and priorities (e.g. HighScope, 2020; Dodd-Nufrio, 2011; Edwards, 2002). Similarly, teachers and teacher candidates tend to align with different approaches and view their role in the classroom in many different ways. Teacher candidates have different views about the most important goals of early childhood education programs; some of those goals might be easier to develop online than others. This way, teachers' views might shape their respective online experiences.

Lastly, while online programs might not be sufficient to train early childhood educators, a combination of online and remote learning might be an effective way of training early childhood teachers. However, little research addresses the preference for format in early childhood. Lastly, biases exist about the effectiveness of online early childhood teacher preparation; students' perspectives need to be taken into account when making recommendations. This study aims to explore these issues by answering the following research questions:

1. What format has best helped teacher candidates acquire the key competencies of early childhood educators as outlined by NAEYC? What learning modality has best-helped teacher candidates stay engaged in their learning?
2. Given a choice, what is the ideal instructional modality for teacher candidates in early childhood: in-person, online, or a combination of both? Was this preference similar for candidates seeking different degrees (such as graduate or undergraduate)?
3. How important is it to build social connections and social networks for early childhood teacher candidates during their training? Are candidates who value the social aspects of their training more likely to prefer an in-person education?

4. What do teachers view as the most important goal(s) in early childhood education? Are these views related to their preference between online and in-person instruction?

Method

Participants

The participants for this study were 101 college students working towards a degree in early childhood education. Participants were drawn from two large universities in a large metropolitan city in the Northwestern U.S. All participants were enrolled in spring semester 2020 coursework preparing them to work with young children. All participants had taken in-person courses to prepare them to become teachers. In the middle of this semester, all courses had shifted to online instruction due to the novel COVID-19 health crisis. Table 3.1 describes the degree students were seeking; 47 participants were working towards an associate's degree, 16 were working towards a BS or BA degree, and 38 were working towards a master's degree. The largest number of respondents were working toward an AS.

Participants	*n*	%
Degree Working Toward:		
AS	47	46.5
BS/BA	16	15.8
MA	38	37.6
Total	101	100.0

Table 3.1 *Description of Participants*

Instrument and Procedure

Participants were recruited by faculty in the early childhood education courses they were enrolled in during the spring semester of 2020. Participants were notified that participation was fully voluntary, and they all signed consent forms. All participants were asked to fill out a short online survey. The survey was designed especially for this study by the study authors. A small group of students reviewed the survey before it was administered to make sure the questions addressed their experiences.

The survey attempted to tap into the following constructs:

- learning modality that has best helped teacher candidates acquire the key competencies of early childhood educators as outlined by NAEYC;
- learning modality that has best-helped teacher candidates stay engaged in their learning;
- ideal instruction format for teacher candidates, given a choice;
- importance of social interactions and networking as part of their higher education experience; and
- early childhood education goals prioritized by teacher candidates.

Item by item description of the instrument is presented in the result section.

Results

The data were analyzed in SPSS using descriptive statistics. The first research question asked what learning modality has best helped teacher candidates acquire the key competencies of early childhood educators as outlined by NAEYC. For each competency, teacher candidates were asked to indicate what learning modality has helped them most; in-person, online, or both equally. Table 3.2 shows the frequencies and percentages for their answers. Most respondents (n = 72, 71.3%) indicated that in-person learning better prepared them "to understand child development." Similarly, most indicated (n = 68, 67.3%) that in-person learning better prepared them "to understand young children's needs." The majority also indicated that "in-person learning better prepared them" for the following: (a) to design a hands-on interactive curriculum (n = 77, 76.2%); (b) to deliver a hands-on interactive curriculum (n = 76, 75.2%); (c) to create supportive learning environments (n = 73, 72.3%); (d) to collaborate with family and other professionals (n = 65, 64.4%); (e) to observe and document young children's learning and development (n = 70, 69.3%); (f) to support young children's social and emotional needs (n = 65, 64.4%); (g) to manage young children's behaviors (n = 71, 70.3%); (h) to address the needs of young children with delays or disabilities (n = 71, 70.3%). Overall, the majority of respondents indicated that an in-person learning modality better prepared them for the classroom. The first research question also explored what learning modality has helped teacher candidates stay most engaged in their learning. The majority (n = 83, 82.2%) felt that in-person learning helped them "feel most engaged in my learning," as described in Table 3.2.

Survey Question: What type of learning modality better-prepared respondents for the following?	*n*	%
Better prepared me to understand child development		
In-person	72	71.3
Combination	28	27.7
Online	1	1.0
Total	101	100.0
Better prepared me to understand young children's needs		
In-person	68	67.3
Combination	30	29.7
Online	3	3.0
Total	101	100.0
Better prepared me to design hands-on interactive curriculum		
In-person	77	76.2
Combination	18	17.8
Online	6	5.9
Total	101	100.0
Better prepared me to deliver hands-on interactive curriculum		
In-person	76	75.2
Combination	21	20.8
Online	4	4.0
Total	101	100.0

Survey Question: What type of learning modality better-prepared respondents for the following?	*n*	%
Better prepared me to create supportive learning environments		
In-person	73	72.3
Combination	23	22.8
Online	5	5.0
Total	101	100.0
Better prepared me to collaborate with family and other professionals		
In-person	65	64.4
Combination	29	28.7
Online	7	6.9
Total	101	100.0
Better prepared me to observe and document young children's learning and development		
In-person	70	69.3
Combination	24	23.8
Online	7	6.9
Total	101	100.0
Better prepared me to support young children's social and emotional needs		
In-person	65	64.4
Combination	30	29.7
Online	6	5.9
Total	101	100.0
Better prepared me to manage young children's behaviors		
In-person	71	70.3
Combination	25	24.8
Online	5	5.0
Total	101	100.0
Better prepared me to address the needs of young children with delays or disabilities		
In-person	71	70.3
Combination	22	21.8
Online	8	7.9
Total	101	100.0

Survey Question: What type of learning modality better-prepared respondents for the following?	*n*	%
Better prepared me to address the needs of young children with delays or disabilities		
In-person	83	82.2
Combination	12	11.9
Online	6	5.9
Total	101	100

Table 3.2 *Learning Modalities and Key Competencies*

The second research question asked what mode of instruction teacher candidates preferred if they were given a choice. Table 3.3 shows that the majority preferred a combination of online and in-person courses as the ideal education format (n = 63, 62.4%); about one in three students preferred all in person (n = 37, 36.6%). Only one respondent (1%) indicated online was the ideal education format.

If I had a choice, my ideal education would be:	*n*	%
In-person	37	36.6
A combination	63	62.4
Online	1	1.0
Total	101	100.0

Table 3.3 *Preferred Learning Modality*

The second research question also asked whether there was a difference in preferred learning modality among candidates seeking different degrees. Chi-square tests of association were used to assess the degree of association between degree level and preferred learning modality (in-person versus a combination of online and face-to-face). For the preferred modality, the online category was excluded to meet the assumptions of chi-square analyses. Chi-square assumes a minimum expected sample size of 5 in each category; there was a frequency of 1 for those who chose online as the ideal educational modality. The assumption that all cells have expected counts greater than five was met and all expected cell frequencies were greater than five. Therefore, there was an adequate sample size to run the chi-square test of association. There was no statistically significant association between degree working toward (AS, BS/BA, MA) and ideal education format, $x^2(2) = 2.97, p = .22$.

The third research question asked how important it was to build social connections and networks to early childhood candidates, and whether candidates who value the social aspects of their training are more likely to prefer an in-person education. Most teacher candidates felt that being able to socialize and/or network in person with others was very important (n = 66, 65.3%). Table 3.4 summarizes these results. In addition, a one-way ANOVA test was performed to see if those candidates who prioritize social interactions also prefer in-person instruction. The results of the one-way ANOVA were significant [F (98,2) = 6.65 p = .002] and showed that those candidates who preferred in-person instruction had the highest scores for valuing social interactions and networking; this was followed by the candidates who preferred a combination of in-person and online. Only one candidate preferred online instruction and had the lowest scores for valuing social interactions. This is summarized in Table 3.5.

One important goal for me in my education experience is being able to socialize and/or network in person with others	n	%
Not important	2	2.0
A little important	5	5.0
Somewhat important	28	27.7
Very important	66	65.3
Total	101	100.0

Table 3.4 *Importance of Social Interactions and Networking*

Preferred Learning Modality	*Scores for Importance of Social Interactions*
All in-person (n = 37)	3.81
A combination (n = 63)	3.44
All online (n = 1)	2.00

Table 3.5 *Scores for Importance of Social Interactions by Preferred Learning Modality*

Lastly, the fourth research question asked what teacher candidates viewed as the most important goal(s) in early education. This is summarized in Figure 1. Table 3.6 shows the frequencies and percentages of teachers' ratings of what they thought were the most important goals of early childhood education. Most teachers felt that play and exploration were most important (n = 72, 71.3) followed by the following goals:

- Learn to regulate emotions (n = 49, 48.5% rated as most important)
- Friendships and social skills (n = 48, 47.5% rated as most important)
- Language and vocabulary (n = 48, 47.5% rated as most important)
- School readiness/academic skills (n = 39, 36.6% rated as most important)

Survey Question: As a teacher, I think the most important goal of early childhood education is:	n	%
Play and exploration		
Least important	10	9.9
Not so important	2	2.0
Important	8	7.9
Very important	9	8.9
Most important	72	71.3
Total	101	100.0
Learn to regulate emotions		
Least important	7	6.9
Not so important	9	8.9
Important	13	12.9

Survey Question: As a teacher, I think the most important goal of early childhood education is:	*n*	%
Very important	23	22.8
Most important	49	48.5
Total	101	100.0
Friendships and social skills		
Least important	3	3.0
Not so important	9	8.9
Important	11	10.9
Very important	30	29.7
Most important	48	47.5
Total	101	100.0
Language and vocabulary		
Least important	6	5.9
Not so important	14	13.9
Important	12	11.9
Very important	21	20.8
Most important	48	47.5
Total	101	100.0
School readiness/academic skills		
Least important	16	15.8
Not so important	14	13.9
Important	12	11.9
Very important	20	19.8
Most important	39	38.6
Total	101	100.0

Table 3.6 *Goals and Priorities in Early Childhood*

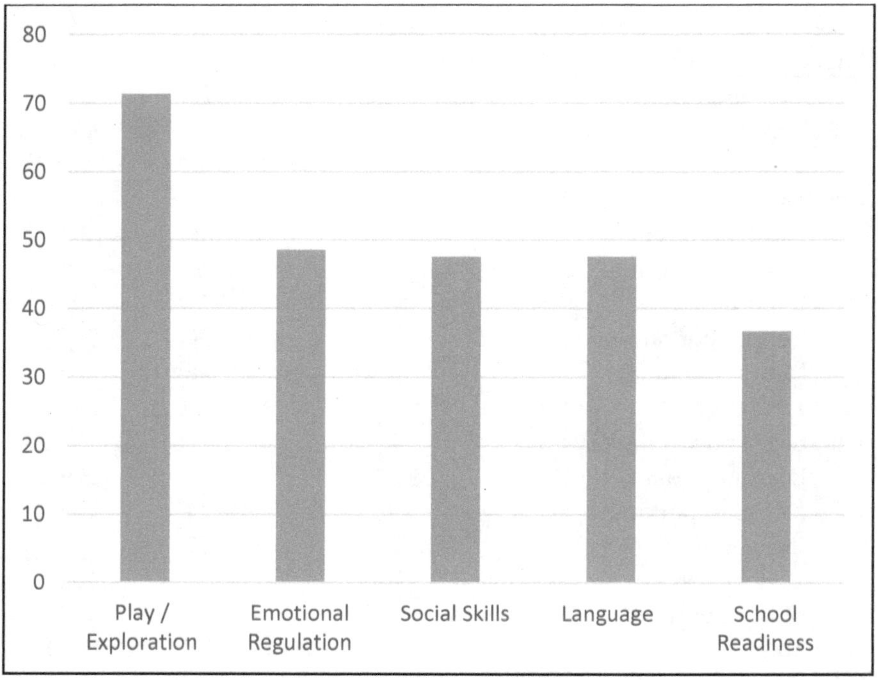

Figure 1. *Teacher's Most Important Goals in Early Childhood Education*

Question four also asked whether teachers' views of the most important goals of early childhood education were related to their preference for in-person, combination, or online instruction. A MANOVA test was performed to compare if teacher candidates in each of the three groups (prefers in-person instruction, combination, or online) scored their goals differently. The results were not statistically significant (Wilk's Lambda = .88, $p = .26$), indicating that teachers' goals did not affect their preferred learning modality.

Discussion

The COVID-19 health crisis presented the opportunity to study whether in fact, young adults consider the online environment optimal for their career preparation. Higher education institutions have been shifting coursework to remote learning in the past years (Govindarajan & Srivastava, 2020). This shift is expected to continue to grow, even after the health crisis has been overcome. This study proposes that the opinions of teacher candidates should help inform this shift.

Early childhood educators value interdisciplinary, hands-on, collaborative learning that stresses exploration and social interactions. For these reasons, early childhood candidates were thought to be less inclined to favor an online learning environment. Similarly, the competencies to become an effective early childhood educator might not be easily achieved in an online environment.

Preferred Learning Modalities

The results of this study have indicated that an overwhelming number of early childhood teachers favored the in-person learning format, expressing that all the key competencies for early childhood educators were better acquired in person. Similarly, the majority felt that the in-person environment helped them stay engaged in learning.

The results have also shown that if given the choice, the majority of candidates prefer a combination of online and in-person learning options. Nevertheless, one in three candidates preferred the all in-person option. Only one candidate preferred to complete a degree entirely online. These findings should be regarded as highly informative when making decisions regarding delivery modes for teacher preparation programs. Despite the assumption that most young adults would prefer to obtain their degrees online (Lederman, 2020), only one candidate indicated this option was the first choice.

Moreover, the results have shown that this preference did not differ among candidates seeking different degrees. The assumption was that undergraduate students would have valued in-person learning because of the social experiences. At the same time, the assumption also was that graduate students would have preferred the online or combination options since they would have been more focused on professional preparation than on social experiences. Yet, these assumptions did not play out and the preference for a combination of an in-person and online experience was uniform across education levels.

Social Interactions as Part of the Learning Experience

Another major finding of this study was that the ability to socialize and network in person with other people constituted a very important component of most students' higher education experience. In addition, the extent to which students considered the ability to build social connections and networks to be very important was related to their preferred learning modality. Thus, students who chose in-person education as their preferred learning modality also tended to have the highest scores in responses to questions regarding social interactions.

Teachers' Goals

The findings have shown that teacher candidates found play and exploration to be their most important goals in early childhood education, whereas school readiness and academic skills were the least important. The assumption was that teachers who valued play and exploration more would have been more likely to prefer in-person learning modalities than teachers who have valued academic skills since academic skills are easier to develop online. Nevertheless, these goals did not impact teacher candidate choice for in-person or online learning. Teachers uniformly chose the combination option.

Conclusion: Lessons for the Future

These tumultuous times have given us the opportunity to learn lessons that might serve higher education institutions offering early childhood teacher preparation programs in the future. Students don't feel that the online environment is adequate to form them as early childhood educators and achieve the key competencies in their field. They do not want to shift their education online, but they do appreciate a combination of online and in-person options. Teacher candidates see their ability to socialize and develop professional networks as an important part of their education; as one teacher candidate expressed "Online classes are not as effective, because they lack the environment of being among many like-minded teachers motivated to grow in our profession." Institutions should consider teacher candidate preferences as they design programs in these new circumstances.

References

Dodd-Nufrio, A. T. (2011). Reggio Emilia, Maria Montessori, and John Dewey: Dispelling teachers' misconceptions and understanding theoretical foundations. *Early Childhood Education Journal, 39*(4), 235-237.

Edwards, C.P. (2002). Three approaches from Europe: Waldorf, Montessori and Reggio Emilia. *Early Childhood Research and Practice, 4* (1). http://ecrp.uiuc.edu/v4n1/edwards.html.

Govindarajan, V., & Srivastava, A. (2020). What the Shift to Virtual Learning Could Mean for the Future of Higher Ed. https://hbr.org/2020/03/what-the-shift-to-virtual-learning-could-mean-for-the-future-of-higher-ed

HighScope. Head Start Alignment. (2020). https://highscope.org/our-reach/head-start/

Lederman, D. (2019, June 5). Inside Higher Ed. https://www.insidehighered.com/digital-learning/article/2019/06/05/annual-survey-shows-online-college-students-increasingly

National Association for the Education of Young Children. (2019). Professional Competencies and Standards for Early Childhood Educators. https://www.naeyc.org/sites/default/files/globally-shared/downloads/PDFs/resources/position-statements/professional_standards_and_competencies_for_early_childhood_educators.pdf.

Piaget, J. (1972). *To Understand Is to Invent.* New York: The Viking Press, Inc.

Vygotsky, L. S. (1978). *Mind in society: The development of higher psychological processes.* Cambridge, MA: Harvard University Press.

Section II

Diverse Early Childhood Experiences in the U.S.

Chapter 4
The Effects of COVID-19 on Socio-Dramatic Play

Tugce Arda-Tuncdemir and Ruth Guirguis

The COVID-19 pandemic has brought about unprecedented challenges across the globe, affecting every aspect of society, including early childhood education. As educators and caregivers have strived to adapt to the evolving circumstances, one critical area of concern has been the impact of the pandemic on play in early childhood education. Play is not just a fun activity for young children; primarily, dramatic play is fundamental to their development, fostering creativity, social skills, and emotional intelligence. This chapter explores the effects of COVID-19 on children's play, strategies to support play during the pandemic, and the long-term implications for the field.

Defining Play

Young children acquire much of their knowledge in the early years through play, which makes play imperative and a tool for learning during these years. Specifically, play facilitates general and skill-based learning, creative thinking, and self-esteem and encourages divergent thinking (Johnson et al., 2005). Sutton-Smith (2016) explains that play mirrors human challenges and the behaviors necessary for survival. Moreover, play not only aids academic achievement in young children but also serves as a means of emotional support during times of crisis (Sutton-Smith, 2016).

The term play is hard to define and articulate, because play is abstract and has multiple meanings for different groups and individuals. According to Vygotsky (1978) play is a vehicle for the child to behave beyond their chronological age. Vygotsky (1978) describes play as having three main components. The first is the ability for a child to create an imaginary situation; second, take on and act out roles; and, lastly, to follow a set of rules that were determined by the roles children took on during play during social or group settings. Hence, play supports much-needed social skills and processes that foster positive social development. The ambiguities of play, specifically the intricate functions between what play entails and the aligned developmental outcomes of play, make defining play challenging. Sutton-Smith (1997) defines play's ambiguities as a progressional function through seven rhetorics: developmental play, risky play, sports play, cultural play, imaginary play, solitary play, and frivolous play. Moreover, play is existential, simple, complex, and "characterized by dualities that are genetic, affective, performative, experiential, and culturally relative" (Sutton-Smith, 2008, p.118).

There are different types of play in which children participate in during their younger years. Parten (1933) has described the following developmental stages in play:

1. Solitary play: Solitary is when a child plays alone and is entirely absorbed in their activities. It is common in infants and toddlers who have not yet developed social play skills.
2. Parallel Play: In parallel play, children play alongside each other but do not actively interact or share toys. This type of play is often seen in toddlers and is an early step toward more social forms of play.
3. Associative Play: In associative play, children begin to interact with each other while playing. They may share toys or materials but do not have a defined structure or goal for their play. This type of play is common in preschoolers.
4. Cooperative Play: Cooperative play involves children working together in organized and structured activities. They have a common goal, assigned roles, and follow rules. Board games and team sports are examples of cooperative play.

Socio-Dramatic Play is a specific type of play that involves children taking on roles and engaging in pretend scenarios. It is a form of imaginative play where children use their creativity and social skills to act out situations, often inspired by real-life experiences or stories they have encountered. Most of the time, socio-dramatic play is cooperative, as it requires complex negotiations about role assignments and narratives. Socio-dramatic play is an activity in which children learn to interact with one another in acceptable ways in social contexts established by society, culture, and history. It is the extent of the social competence that a preschool child holds that can be used as an indicator of school readiness (Mathieson & Banerjee, 2010).

Dramatic Play and Socio-emotional Development

The present chapter focuses on socio-dramatic play in preschool children. Explicitly, role-playing socio-dramatic play allows children to understand and interact with others in various scenarios, where they develop empathy and gain a deeper understanding of different perspectives and roles in real life. Consequently, socio-dramatic play can also help children learn about and understand different cultures, traditions, and societal roles as they mimic various professions and activities. Lastly, socio-dramatic play nurtures children's social and emotional regulation by developing language to express themselves and learning to negotiate and cooperate with peers.

While young children engage in both structured and unstructured play in school settings, during unstable times, and when required to be at home while social distancing, the type of play children carry out serves as a vehicle children can use to navigate their thoughts and fears and manage feelings. Consequently, the focus of play as a means of expressing and coping during a crisis should be a continuum effort between the school and home setting. Adjusting how, when, and who can scaffold children's play during challenging times is imperative to create and develop a safe space for play and the processes and skills it supports. Preschool children participating in associative and cooperative play will return to independent play. Accordingly, it is essential that during independent play, aspects of both dramatic and pretend play are embedded and emphasized for young children to learn to process some of the emotions, as dramatic and pretend play can support key emotional processes children need to manage within a different environment and when faced with anxieties and fears.

Play serves as a mechanism for survival during times of crisis (Sutton-Smith, 2016). Sutton-Smith (2016) proposed six distinct play forms, which allow children to convey different emotions and modify their emotional state to meet the demands set by the current environment. Sutton-Smith's (2016) framework suggests that shock, fear, loneliness, happiness, anger, and disgust align with six main play forms. Those play forms, respectively, are teasing and hazing, games of risk-taking, festivals, peak experiences, contests, nonsense, and profanity. These play formats create a platform for specific types of play behavior to be displayed by young children. The functions of these behaviors have a positive and real-world application to young children's living environments. For example, Sutton-Smith (2016) suggests that behaviors such as teasing allow for the development of resilience, risk-taking allows for a sense of courage to be developed, and contests can lead to vigilance. These processes help young children adapt and thrive during isolation and unfamiliar circumstances. These key skills can be observed in dramatic and pretend play.

Younger children often find it easier to work with their anxieties and emotions symbolically, as this is a form of communication that is familiar to them. According to Korat et al. (2003), most researchers of children's pretend play have linked social competence, socially appropriate behaviors, and mental processes through role play (Roskos & Christie, 2001; Tsao, 2008; Vygotsky, 1978). Children imitate behaviors and feelings that they observe. This process of observation and imitation results from the child acquiring contextual meaning through play, which is then needed in the development of metacognition. Contextual meaning influences how children begin to think about their thinking and understand and interpret what is happening around them. Dramatic play allows young children to express their thoughts and feelings without relying on their limited expressive vocabulary to communicate their needs and concerns. During a crisis, dramatic play can help young children to make sense of their current home situations, as children can create a narrative and engage in the cause and effects of being at home without the ability to see and play with classmates. This type of play can be supported by engaging children through art, puppets, storytime, and role-playing.

Families play a key role in facilitating children's play, and a family's cultural background can impact the amount and type of play young children choose (Gosso & Carvalho, 2013). For example, some families believe that elicit and active play is messy and loud. When families share spaces and older members co-exist, some play activities that are considered loud or disruptive are discouraged. Religious practices also play a role in the type of play that is encouraged. During times of religious practices, families may choose for the play to cease or take a more structured form. Families' perspectives on "right" and "wrong" types of play shape what and how children decide to engage in play and playful activities. Families may consider active play to be wrong when a child is indoors, hence limiting the time young children devote to active play.

Similarly, parental involvement is also based on families' practices and perspectives of play (Gosso & Carvalho, 2013). Some families may engage in play with young children, while others delegate the role of play to be carried out by siblings. These approaches differ as they either allow young children to have adult-child interactions or peer-sibling interactions, shaping the type of play planning, skills, and language used during play with different members. However, it is critical to note the importance of adult interactions during play in order to observe and scaffold it.

The Effects of the Lack of Socio-Dramatic Play

The COVID-19 pandemic caused significant challenges for schools and child care centers worldwide. Due to lockdowns and social distancing measures, many early childhood education facilities had to close, leaving parents and educators struggling to find a safe and effective learning environment for young children. Additionally, children faced restrictions on accessing playgrounds and public parks and had to follow gathering restrictions and quarantine requirements.

During this time of increased stress and worry, children also faced reduced access to play and its benefits for their development and coping. Play is one of the most essential ways to support psychological and physical health and helps children cope with stress, anxiety, and trauma (Chatterjee, 2018). It provides stability, normalcy, and enjoyment, making it crucial for children's overall well-being. Yet, the COVID-19 pandemic had a significant impact on socio-dramatic play among children, primarily due to the public health measures and restrictions put in place to reduce the spread of the virus.

Play Vignette: Deniz and Demir

The following vignette explores several of the challenges experienced by children during the COVID-19 pandemic. This vignette is based on the authors' personal and professional experience and illustrates the available research on play experiences during the pandemic.

During the spring of 2020, two kids spent their time playing in their backyard. Since schools were closed and social distancing was required, their backyard became their playground, classroom, and safe space from the uncertainties of the world. The elder child, Deniz, was known for being social, talkative, and enthusiastic, and his younger brother, Demir, followed his lead. While they played, parents watched them from a safe distance to ensure their safety while allowing them to explore. One April morning, after playing soccer, riding bikes, and observing a bug, Deniz asked when he could invite his neighbors to play in their backyard. All the kids on their street played in their own backyards but talked to each other from a distance. It was tough for the kids to understand why they could not play together, and even parents did not know when the pandemic would end. After discussing COVID-19 safety with Deniz, his mother found him playing tag with his friends in their neighbor's backyard. She reminded him of the precautions, and he replied, "Mom, we're not touching each other. We're tagging each other with small sticks." They had already figured out a way to play together while remaining physically distant.

Vignette Analysis: Changes to Play Experienced During the Pandemic

The example above highlights the way young children develop resilience through play. Imperative to the interrelation between play and psychological underpinning is the development of resilience. Resilience is better defined as overcoming challenges and one's adaptability to adversity that leads to positive developmental outcomes. Play allows children to reduce the many stresses they face while learning new skills. Specifically, play allows children to problem solve, manage strong feelings, express thoughts and feelings verbally and non-verbally, and develop confidence in their abilities (UNCESCO, 2019).

In addition, the vignette above explores several of the challenges and changes experienced by young children and their families when attempting to play during the pandemic. Most children confronted several obstacles.

Changes to Play: Social Distancing, Play Spaces, and Play Themes

One of the most profound impacts of the pandemic was the need for social distancing and isolation. Children were often separated from their peers, which limited opportunities for group play, including socio-dramatic play. Playdates, group activities, and in-person school experiences were disrupted. Similarly, play areas when families were sheltering in place had sometimes been a struggle. Lack of space for children to move and explore have caused young children to disengage in creative play. Sharing common spaces with other parents, siblings, and/or extended family members during shelter-in-place rules can reduce the freedom of expression and active play, which plays a role in impulse control/emotional regulation (Rimm-Kaufman & Wanless, 2012). Furthermore, time for play and time to plan for play can also be a barrier to pretend and imaginary play. Families have needed to focus on issues of safety, shelter, and food, as well as financial burdens; these factors played a role in limiting the time that families had to devote to young children's play needs and have constrained much-needed time for co-planning for play and observing play in young children. Lastly, the pandemic has brought about changes in children's play themes, and some children incorporated pandemic-related themes into their dramatic play, such as pretending to be doctors or nurses treating "patients." This illustrates the way play helps children process their experiences, and it also reflects the influence of the pandemic on play.

Planning for Changes in Play and Play Spaces

Understanding the function play has on alleviating levels of toxic stress is as important as understanding some barriers that prevent creating optimal play scenarios during isolation. Acknowledging the challenges and barriers during a crisis can help families accommodate appropriate places and spaces for play. Fostering dramatic and pretend play requires caregivers and families to provide an uninterrupted setting for various themes and props that support each theme (Pratt Prairie, 2013). During a crisis, finding a space to allow for uninterrupted play is not necessarily feasible. The themes and props may also not be something families have access to; they also may not have familiarity with setting up thematic play spaces.

Taking time to plan for play is perhaps more important than the play itself. The process of play planning develops representational skills as well as cognitive control (Pratt Prairie, 2013). Cognitive controls allow children to follow and comply with rules, manage emotions, and carry out problem-solving tasks on their own (Bronson, 2000). These skills are of particular importance to young children entering formal schooling. Nevertheless, planning may be a factor that has been difficult for many families faced with many responsibilities. Planning, themes, and materials for play are just a few barriers that can challenge the notion of an optimal play scenario. There are external factors that present themselves during a crisis that families and caregivers need to address, and optimal play situations are only sometimes feasible. Many social factors within families and communities contribute to play inequities among young children.

Changes in Play Platforms: Virtual Play

Virtual learning significantly changed early childhood education throughout the pandemic. Teachers offered interactive games, educational apps, and virtual storytimes to keep young learners engaged and connected to their peers and teachers. Caregivers were also advised to organize supervised video chats and phone calls for their children and friends. However, educators and parents needed help finding resources and materials for their kids to play or otherwise engage with.

Several educators organized virtual play sessions for parents and teachers. For example, the first author has organized such sessions in Turkey and the United States. These events focused on interactive play and included information on how to facilitate play with children. The sessions consisted of caregivers and educators listening to information about the importance of play, play development, and play examples. They were asked to bring everyday materials to the sessions (such as stones, sticks, cooking pots, utensils, beans, fabrics, and lids). They explored self-regulated play using the materials they brought. They discussed what they played, how they felt during their playtime, and shared indoor and outdoor play ideas. These virtual meetings helped them practice mindfulness, creativity, social and emotional awareness, and improvisation during physical distancing. The participants were able to guide the process with young children. This example highlights the importance of supporting play in virtual contexts. While virtual play sessions do not replace traditional play, these sessions help attendees understand the importance of play and socializing during the pandemic.

Lessons Learned and Implications for Practice

The COVID-19 pandemic compelled early childhood education to adjust quickly, highlighting the resourcefulness and inventiveness of teachers and guardians. Despite the significant obstacles, educators gained valuable insights that have the potential to influence the future of early childhood education.

Following the pandemic, the significance of being flexible, adaptable, and integrating technology in early childhood education has become more evident than ever. Play still lies at the core of early childhood development, but the manner in which it is facilitated may continue to change, merging traditional techniques with inventive approaches.

It is essential to remember that the principles of early childhood education and play remain constant. Despite the difficulties, the dedication to giving young children the best possible foundation for their future should always inform practices. This ensures children have the necessary resources to succeed in an ever-evolving world.

Lessons For Teachers

The pandemic has brought about significant changes for teachers, providing valuable lessons and implications for play-based learning in the future. These insights have influenced how educators approach play-based learning and expand our knowledge of the critical role play takes in child development.

Teachers have shown exceptional adaptability and creativity during the pandemic by finding innovative ways to engage children in play despite remote or socially distanced learning challenges, such as virtual playrooms, virtual field trips, interactive storytelling, Google G-Suites, Google Hangouts, and Conceptual Playworld (Ahmad & Zabadi, 2020; Goldschmidt, 2020; Fleer, 2020). They have also learned to use digital tools and platforms to enhance play-based learning.

The COVID-19 pandemic has highlighted the importance of play in promoting children's mental health and well-being (Graber et al., 2021). Teachers have recognized how play can reduce stress and anxiety and will continue incorporating play-based strategies to support emotional growth and resilience (O'Keeffe & McNally, 2021). Even in virtual settings, teachers have observed how play can bring students together, emphasizing the need to maintain these connections through play.

Building a playful pathway towards resilience in children requires active engagement and scaffolding from educators and primary caregivers. More importantly, this playful pathway will allow young children to develop a sense of efficacy and control over their immediate environment. Building resilience in children is a form of a "mediating process that addresses a functional domain in a child's development and enhances it. A pathway to resilience can be described as a process that is supportive of a child's healthy holistic development" (UNESCO, 2019, p. 15).

Play as a pathway to resilience provides young children with active play participation from adults, adult modeling of positive social behaviors, a sense of autonomy and independence, and enabling children's ability to regulate their stress by reducing toxic stress (UNESCO, 2019). Moreover, play as a pathway to building resilience will restore self-empowerment in children by giving them the opportunity to develop the life skills they need to thrive as adults.

In the future, teachers should continue to participate in professional development opportunities to improve their play practice and socio-emotional skills. They should also expand their understanding of the impact of play on learning outcomes and increase the use of evidence-based practices to inform their teaching.

Lessons for Parents

Throughout the COVID-19 pandemic, parents have also demonstrated incredible adaptability and creativity in encouraging play and learning at home (Garbe et al., 2020). One crucial aspect to consider is monitoring and regulating technology usage to ensure it complements, rather than replaces, play experiences. Although virtual playdates have been encouraged, the pandemic has increased reliance on digital devices, highlighting the need for parents to balance screen time with active and imaginative play (Egan et al., 2020).

Therefore, amidst this pandemic, parents aimed to provide opportunities for children to explore and engage with the natural world (Moore et al., 2020). Engaging with nature allows children to explore and learn, fostering independence and creativity. The therapeutic effects of play have been shown to reduce stress and anxiety, benefiting not only children but also parents. Play should continue to be a valuable tool for promoting family well-being and bonding.

Lessons for Administrators

The educational and recreational play practices have been affected by the COVID-19 pandemic, and administrators have learned valuable lessons. These lessons can guide policy-making and decision-making to create more effective, resilient, and inclusive play environments in the post-pandemic era.

Administrators have realized the importance of adaptability and resilience when facing unforeseen disruptions (Jalongo, 2021). There is a need to to change the play practices in response to changing circumstances to ensure continuity and quality in play-based experiences. These experiences should prioritize inclusivity, equity, and access to all participants, accommodating their diverse needs and backgrounds (Ciuffetelli Parker & Conversano, 2021).

The pandemic has also accelerated technology integration into play practices, and administrators should continue exploring how digital tools and platforms can enhance play-based learning and recreational activities while ensuring equitable access. The sense of connection and social support fostered by play can contribute to stronger communities, and administrators should focus on this aspect (Inderawati et al., 2023). There is a need to reinforce resources for data collection, analysis, and research partnerships to inform evidence-based decision-making and establish contingency plans to ensure the continuity of play-based programs during future crises. These plans should consider various scenarios, including remote and socially distanced play.

Finally, administrators have a crucial role in advocating for the importance of play in child development and securing funding for play programs. They must clearly communicate the benefits of play and its long-term impact to garner stakeholder support. These lessons underscore the enduring value of play as an essential element of human growth and connection.

Conclusion

The COVID-19 pandemic has positively and negatively affected children's play at home. On the one hand, families have had more opportunities to spend time together, which has led to bonding through play and creativity. Parents and caregivers have been using board games, outdoor activities, and imaginative play to keep children engaged and entertained during lockdowns. However, the increased use of digital devices for remote learning and entertainment has raised concerns about excessive screen time and its impact on children's physical and mental health. Finding a balance between screen-based activities and active, unstructured play has become a significant challenge for parents. Overall, the pandemic has highlighted the importance of creating a supportive play environment at home where children can continue to develop essential life skills and maintain their emotional well-being, even during unforeseen disruptions like COVID-19.

The COVID-19 pandemic has had a significant and varied impact on children's play, both at home and in school. Due to widespread school closures and remote learning, children have been unable to enjoy the structured playtime they usually would during recess and physical education classes. The lack of opportunities for social interaction and physical activity has raised concerns regarding the effect on children's overall development. Play is not just a source of joy but also a vital way to develop social skills, problem-solving abilities, and emotional resilience. Safety measures such as mask mandates and physical distancing have also changed the dynamics of play in schools, creating a situation where children have had to adjust to new norms and limitations in their interactions with their peers. These changes highlight the need for schools to find creative ways to prioritize play in the curriculum, even during ongoing or future health challenges.

In the post-COVID era, it is crucial for administrators and policymakers to create an inclusive and adaptable play environment for all children (International Literacy Centre, 2020). They can achieve this by embracing technology, prioritizing safety, and promoting community engagement. By doing so, they can ensure that play remains an integral part of education and recreation, promoting holistic development and well-being for children. Additionally, it is vital for administrators and policymakers to provide clear guidelines and resources for schools to navigate these unprecedented times. By addressing these issues and valuing play as a crucial component of childhood development, they can mitigate the adverse effects of COVID-19 on children's play and contribute to the overall well-being of the next generation.

References

Ahmad, N. A. A., & Zabadi, A. M. (2020). Transition to Online Education in Palestinian kindergartens During the Coronavirus (COVID-19) Pandemic: Al - Ameen Kindergarten as a Case Study. *American Journal of Educational Research, 8*(8), 600–608.

Bronson, M.B. (2000). *Self-regulation in early childhood.* New York, NY: Guilford Publications.

Chatterjee, S. (2018). Children's coping, adaptation and resilience through play in situations of crisis. Children, *Youth and Environments, 28*(2), 119–145. https://doi.org/10.7721/chilyoutenvi.28.2.0119

Ciuffetelli Parker, D. & Conversano P. (2021). Narratives of Systemic Barriers and Accessibility: Poverty, Equity, Diversity, Inclusion, and the Call for a Post-Pandemic New Normal. *Frontiers in Education, 6.* DOI=10.3389/feduc.2021.704663. https://www.frontiersin.org/articles/10.3389/feduc.2021.704663

Egan, S., M., Beatty, C., & Hoyne, C. (2020). Play-Impact of COVID-19 Restrictions on Young Children's Play Learning and Development: Key findings from the Play and Learning in the Early Years (PLEY) Survey. July 2020. https://www.researchgate.net/publication/342701227_ Play_-_Impact_of_COVID19_Restrictions_on_Young_Children%27s_Play_Learning_and_ Development_Key_Findings_from_the_Play_and_Learning_in_the_Early_Years_PLEY_ Survey_-_Play.

Fleer, M. (2020). Re-imagining play spaces in early childhood education: Supporting girls' motive orientation to STEM in times of COVID-19. *Journal of Early Childhood Research,* 1–8. https://doi.org/10.1177/1476718X20969848.

Garbe, A., Ogurlu, U., Logan, N., & Cook, P. (2020). COVID-19 and Remote Learning: Experiences of Parents with Children during the Pandemic. *American Journal of Qualitative Research,* 4(3), 45-65. https://doi.org/10.29333/ajqr/8471

Goldschmidt, K. (2020). The COVID-19 Pandemic: Technology use to Support the Wellbeing of Children. *J Pediatr Nurs, 53*:88-90. doi: 10.1016/j.pedn.2020.04.013. Epub 2020 Apr 16. PMID: 32317129; PMCID: PMC7161478.

Gosso, Y., & Carvalho, A.M. (2013). Play and Cultural Context.Gosso Y, Almeida Carvalho AM. Play and Cultural Context. *Encyclopedia on Early Childhood Development*. https://www.child-encyclopedia.com/play/according-experts/play-and-cultural-context.

Graber, K.M., Bryne, E.M., Goodacre, E. J., Kirby, N., Kulkarni, K., O'Farrelly, & Ramchandani, P. G. (2021). A rapid review of the impact of quarantine and restricted environments on children's play and the role of play in children's health. *Child Care Health Dev.,47*:143–153. https://doi.org/10.1111/cch.12832

Inderawati, R., Eryansyah, E., Maharrani, D., Suhendi, D., & Siahaan, S. (2023). Virtual drama performance: Is it a need due to pandemic or technological era? *English Review: Journal of English Education, 11*(2), 551-560. https://doi.org/10.25134/erjee.v11i2.6653

International Literacy Centre (2020). *Responding to COVID-19, Briefing Note 3: Resetting educational priorities in challenging times.* London: UCL Institute of Education.

Jalongo, M.R. The Effects of COVID-19 on Early Childhood Education and Care: Research and Resources for Children, Families, Teachers, and Teacher Educators. *Early Child Educ J., 49*(5):763-774. doi: 10.1007/s10643-021-01208-y. Epub 2021 May 24. PMID: 34054286; PMCID: PMC8142069.

Johnson, J.E., Christie, J.F. & Wardle, F. (2005). *Play, development, and early education.* Boston, MA: Pearson Education Inc.

Korat, O., Bahar, E., & Snapir, M. (2002). Sociodramatic play as opportunity for literacy development: The teacher's role. *The Reading Teacher, 56*(4), 386-393.

Mathieson, K., & Banerjee, R. (2010). Pre-school peer play: The beginnings of social competence. *Educational & Child Psychology, 27(1)*, 9-20.

Moore, S.A., Faulkner, G., Rhodes, R.E. *et al.* (2020).Impact of the COVID-19 virus outbreak on movement and play behaviours of Canadian children and youth: a national survey. *Int J Behav Nutr Phys Act* 17, 85. https://doi.org/10.1186/s12966-020-00987-8

O'Keeffe, C. & McNally, S. (2021). 'Uncharted territory': teachers' perspectives on play in early childhood classrooms in Ireland during the pandemic,

European Early Childhood Education Research Journal, 29(1), 79-95, DOI: 10.1080/1350293X.2021.1872668

Parten , M.B. (1932). Social participation among pre-school children . *Journal of Abnormal and Social Psychology* , 27, 243 – 269

Pratt Prairie, A. (2013). Supporting Sociodramatic Play in Ways that Enhance Academic Learning. *Young Children, 68*(2), 62-68.

Rimm-Kaufman, S. E., & Wanless, S.B. (2012). An ecological perspective for understanding the early development of self-regulatory skills, social skills, and achievement. In E. C. Pianta, Barnett, S. M. Sheridan, & L. M. Justice. *Handbook of Early Childhood Education* (pp. 299-323). New York, NY: Guilford Press.

Roskos, K., & Christie, J. (2001). Examining the play–literacy interface: A critical review and future directions. *Journal of Early Childhood Literacy, 1*(1), 59–89. https://doi.org/10.1177/14687984010011004

Sutton-Smith, B. (1997). *The ambiguity of play.* Harvard University Press.

Sutton-Smith, B. (2008). Play theory: A personal journey and new thoughts. *American Journal of Play, 1(1)*, 80–123.

Sutton-Smith, B. (2016). Play for life: Play theory and play as emotional survival. Rochester: Strong Museum of Children's Play.

Tsao, Y.-L. (2008). Using Guided Play to Enhance Children's Conversation, Creativity and Competence in Literacy. *Education, 128*(3), 515–520. https://eric.ed.gov/?id=EJ816928

UNESCO International Institute for Capacity-Building in Africa. (2019).

Vygotsky, L. (1978). *Mind in society: The development of higher psychological processes*. Cambridge, MA: Harvard University Press Publications.

About the Contributing Author:

Tugce Arda Tuncdemir, Ph.D. is an Assistant Professor at Pennsylvania State University Harrisburg. Dr. Arda Tuncdemir earned her Ph.D. from the Curriculum and Instruction Department with an emphasis on Early Childhood Education at Pennsylvania State University. Her research interests are play, creative drama, social-emotional learning, anti-bias education, culturally responsive pedagogy, ethics in early childhood, and teacher education, shared through presentations, book chapters, and journals. She has been awarded the Play Policy and Practice Interest Forum (PPPIF) at National Association for the Education of Young Children (NAEYC) Walter F. Drew Emerging Play Scholar Award 2018 and was the 2022-2023 President of The Association for the Study of Play.

Chapter 5
Young Children's Experiences During COVID-19: The Role of Socio-Economic Status and Immigration

Anna Mantagas and Raquel Plotka

One of the most important factors impacting early childhood education during the COVID-19 pandemic was family socio-economic status (SES). SES is associated with family education level, resources, parental employment, and parental time. SES is also intertwined with a family's immigration status and whether a child is an English language learner. Consequently, the experiences of children from diverse SES backgrounds have differed significantly during the pandemic. In many ways, the pandemic highlighted the gap in opportunities children in the United States experienced before the crisis. This gap in opportunities should help guide future practices and policies.

SES and Education in the United States

Education and income are intricately related in the United States, impacting the learning experiences of young children. For example, family household income and socioeconomic status generally depend on the education level of the heads of the household. According to the 2020 United States Census, the average household income was $67,521. Heads of household with no high school diploma averaged $29,547, those with high school diploma but no college averaged $47,405, those with some college education were closest to the median at $63,653, and those with a bachelor's degree or higher made an average of $106,936 (Shrider et al., 2021). According to the United States Bureau of Labor Statistics, the likelihood of being classified as working poor diminishes as workers attain higher levels of education. About 13% of labor force participants with less than a high school diploma were classified as working poor, compared with 1.3 percent of those with a bachelor's degree and higher" (U.S. Bureau of Labor Statistics, 2022).

Typically, children of lower SES have poorer outcomes in school. Studies have shown that students of lower SES perform about three academic years behind their more advantaged peers; also, compared to high SES students, low SES students tend to score 20-26 percentage points lower (Karoly, 2015; Bradley, 2023). Finally, low SES students are also more likely to be suspended or ejected from the classroom than their more advantaged peers (Bradley, 2023). All these factors illustrate the way children of low SES are academically disadvantaged compared to their more affluent classmates. As early as kindergarten, the achievement gap between low and high SES students becomes glaringly apparent; students from low SES generally enter school at a lower academic level than their peers and spend a good portion of their academic careers attempting to make the same gains as their classmates (Sacks, 2016). This constant game of catch-up ultimately leads to increased dropout rates (7.2% of low SES students compared to 3.6% for middle and 3.9% for high SES students), lower likelihood of college graduation (14% compared to 60%), and a higher likelihood of incarceration (Bradley, 2023).

Statistically, some English learners are also part of low-income households. According to a 2021 Brookings study, about 20% of American schools enroll 75% of the nation's Dual Language Learners (DLL) - with most of these schools being in low-income areas; according to this same study, 37% of the nation's DLLs live in poverty, and 54% of these DLLs have parents that did not attend college (Quintero & Hansen, 2021). In this chapter, DLL refers to children between the ages of birth and five years of age who are learning two languages simultaneously, their home language in addition to English. This means that the schools supporting most of the DLL students in the nation are concentrated in lower-income areas. Whether or not a DLL resides in a lower SES, the availability of academic resources in a school in a lower-income area (or lack thereof) will most likely negatively impact a student learning English. During the pandemic, schools in lower-income areas were not as adequately prepared for remote instruction as those in more affluent communities, as they had fewer resources to work with and less parental engagement (Miller & Williams-Isom, 2021).

The present chapter attempts to explore the experiences of children of diverse socioeconomic status during the pandemic in order to better understand the different trajectories families and children have faced and provide lessons and recommendations for educators and policymakers.

The Role of SES in ECE Children's Experiences During the Pandemic

The following vignettes were designed to illustrate children's experiences during the pandemic, and the way multiple and cumulative factors shaped children's realities in families with different resources and backgrounds. The names, characters, businesses, events, and incidents in these vignettes are the products of the authors' imagination and reflections on collective personal experiences. The vignettes summarize existing research about the role of SES in young children's experiences.

Vignette I

Jean-Michel, Noah, and Ashby live in a small one-bedroom apartment with their mother. She works at a grocery store, sometimes taking double shifts so she can make extra money to make ends meet. They are a family of recent immigrants from Haiti and speak predominantly Haitian Creole in the home. Jean-Michel, the oldest, is in high school, Noah is in middle school, and Ashby just started preschool in September of 2019 - a few short months before schools closed in March 2020 due to the COVID-19 pandemic.

There is only one laptop in the house and generally, Jean-Michel needs to use it since he has to log into each of his classes on Google Classroom and complete assignments for all of his different classes daily. Ashby often hears his older brother apologizing to his teachers for having his camera off during class time because he needs to watch his little brothers and help them with their homework.

Ashby and Noah have to share Jean-Michel's iPhone to log in and complete their assignments or activities; generally, the middle brother sacrifices his working time to let Ashby see his friends on the small phone screen for a couple of hours a day. Noah barely logs into Zoom at all, because he is helping Ashby log in, complete activities, and interact with his classmates virtually.

Ashby is usually only supervised by his older siblings and often has to stay in the bedroom with Noah; while they are attempting to complete school work in there, Jean-Michel stays in the living room, their mother's sleeping area, closest to the modem where the connection to the neighbor's internet connection is the strongest - something many students of lower SES with minimal access to internet had to do during the pandemic (McClain et al., 2021).

In the few hours of the day that Ashby sees his mother, she is often tired or busy preparing food for the next few days so the boys can eat while she is gone. There is limited interaction between Ashby and his mother, and any at all is far from stimulating or educational; their conversation is usually a series of questions about his day and whether he was a good boy while his brothers were watching him. She does not check his assignments, instead deferring to his two older brothers to do it if they have time because she still is not fluent in written English.

Vignette II

Sara and her older brother, Joey, live in a five-bedroom house complete with a pool and a fully furnished guest bedroom. Their parents work remotely; their father is in technology and data analysis, and their mother is a 15-year teacher in one of the most elite districts in the area. Each member of the family has a personal laptop and the newest iPad or iPhone.

Sara is in kindergarten, while her older brother is in 5th grade. On Mondays, they each work independently in their own rooms using their own personal laptops while their parents regularly check in on each of them. On Tuesdays and Wednesdays, their mother hosts a learning pod in the family room for three other families in the neighborhood that also attend the school in Sara's district (Moyer, 2020); she supervises the kids while she does her own work, though they generally work and interact with one another (and have a great time doing so). On Thursdays and Fridays, Sara attends a learning pod at her friend's house down the street.

Sara regularly interacts with her teacher online and engages in lessons with her peers on screen and with her learning pod. There is always an adult to answer any questions she may have; sometimes, her teacher even rotates through the different learning pods in the neighborhood and hosts them live from the different homes so students can have a turn seeing their teacher in person.

When Sara and Joey end their school day, their parents are not far behind in completing their own work from their respective home offices. They are often able to have dinner together and talk about the day's events, ask their questions, and get help with any homework they have. After dinner, Sara sits with her dad in his office to complete any outstanding assignments, while her older brother sits with their mother in her office to do his.

Vignette Analysis

The cases of Ashby and Sara illustrate both ends of the economic spectrum and represent common cases across multiple homes in the United States and the world during the COVID-19 pandemic. While lower-income families struggled to stay afloat, those with the means were able to benefit from the advent of new programs created specifically for online learning that evolved during this time, such as learning pods (Moyer, 2020).

Students of lower socioeconomic status were more negatively impacted by the COVID-19 pandemic, whereas their more affluent peers had more opportunities for individualized learning. Heads of lower socioeconomic households often had to work outside the home and provide for their families, as there was usually no remote option for their jobs; some even experienced language barriers, housing issues, or job loss (Krogstad et al., 2020). Wealthier families not only had the resources and education to supervise their children during remote learning, but they were generally also more able to afford the support, technology, and space for their children to learn. These factors resulted in an even larger learning gap between students of lower socioeconomic backgrounds and those in more privileged circumstances, then there was before the pandemic. Though online learning was not ideal for most early childhood students, those coming from families with more financial resources were more likely to become active agents of their own learning.

The Experience of ECE Low-SES Children and Their Families

Children in low-income families struggled more educationally due to a lack of parental presence or involvement. Parents were often not home to help their children with homework because people of lower socioeconomic status did not have jobs that could easily be switched to a remote platform (Baska, 2020). Those who lost their jobs often had to hunt for new ones to survive. Consequently, during the pandemic the overarching expectation in families of lower socioeconomic status was that older siblings would take on the household and caretaking responsibilities while the parents would work to financially support their children (Wikle et al., 2018). With parents working, older children had to function as their younger siblings' child care and teachers alike. Naturally, older siblings are not certified educators; though they may have had experience with the same subjects (and even the same teachers and classes as well), they are not pedagogically experienced to serve as the foundation for the early childhood education of their siblings. Giving this responsibility to older siblings while also expecting them to complete their own remote school work was a heavy burden for older siblings to bear - one which directly impacted their respective younger siblings during those formative early childhood years.

Furthermore, families with lower socioeconomic status tended to have limited space, resources, and technology compared to families of higher socioeconomic status. Children need space to learn, play, and explore, especially in the early childhood years (Bodrova & Leong, 2003). It was very hard for students to engage in interactive lessons when they were confined between the four walls of small apartments.

Another issue that emerged during this time was the lack of reliable internet access, which made it difficult for early childhood students to log in and interact with their teachers and peers (Frost, 2021). Similarly, families with multiple siblings did not always have one device per child; usually, the older child with the most assignments and more taxing work would use the available device, while the younger sibling would often either have to share or be left with nothing to use at all (Vogels, 2020).

The lack of internet access and technology, the only real outlet to the outside world during several months of the pandemic, contributed to severe academic regression for early childhood students (Betthäuser et al., 2023). Upon the return to school, teachers saw an abundance of behavioral issues, a lack of stamina for extended periods of reading and writing, and screen dependence. Young children also were functioning at a lower grade level in math and reading than they were before the pandemic (Mantagas, 2023). Though children of lower socioeconomic status have always suffered from achievement gaps due to the aforementioned limitations, the pandemic exacerbated them because young children were not able to have the great equalizer - access to a quality education in a school setting.

The Experience of ECE Higher-SES Children and Their Families

The experience of low-SES children contrasts with the experience of their more affluent peers. Children in more financially stable families may not have made the same academic gains during the pandemic, but they did have more opportunities for success. Higher socioeconomic status and higher education are often positively correlated because wealthier families are more likely to be educated and have a breadth of resources (Shrider et al., 2021). They are more likely to be innovative when it comes to their child's education. Because wealthier families have the funds to do so, some parents were even willing and able to pay for private education in independent schools that remained open during the pandemic (Pandey, 2021).

Parents of higher SES are more likely to be heavily involved in their children's growth and are aware that their respective children's development would be hindered if they did not immerse themselves in their children's education (Bowles, 2018). As a result, multiple parents in communities around the United States created learning pods with small groups of students in the same neighborhood that rotated between different households (Moyer, 2020). These were created for students to maintain the social interactions important to early childhood development and for parents to take turns supervising children while others took that time to work.

Wealthier families also had more spacious homes with workable spaces for home offices, while siblings usually did not even have to share rooms with one another and could work independently in their own spaces. While for families of lower socioeconomic status, online learning may have been a big adjustment, many wealthy families already had the experience of remote work and access to technology - and were, therefore, able to more easily transition to the virtual learning environment the pandemic demanded (Mays & Long, 2020).

Access to reliable internet and technology differed significantly among children and families from different SES backgrounds. For example, many families of higher socioeconomic status had trustworthy internet connections and already had multiple devices in the home pre-pandemic (Vogels, 2020). In his 2021 study for the Joint Center for Housing Studies at Harvard University, Frost explains "...there were many disparities among households with school-age children. Among these households in 2019, 29 percent of those earning less than $30,000 lacked high-speed internet, compared to 23 percent of those earning $30,000-44,999, 18 percent of those earning $45,000-$74,999, and 10 percent of those earning $75,000 or more. Having access does not necessarily remove all obstacles, however. A Pew Research Center survey conducted in April 2020 found that nearly two-thirds of lower-income parents reported that their children would face digital obstacles with schoolwork during the pandemic. Clearly, the higher the household income, the less likely a child will face digital obstacles (Frost, 2021).

Lastly, people with higher education levels also tend to have the ability to work remotely (Hess, 2019); this has played a big role in the ability of parents to spend time with their children during the pandemic when schools closed while also allowing them to keep their jobs and support their families.

The Unique Experiences of Immigrant Children and Their Families

The role of SES in the U.S. is deeply intertwined with immigration status. This is especially true for children in undocumented immigrant families, who experienced the most challenges during the pandemic.

For example, a recent study conducted in 2017 showed that most undocumented immigrants worked in jobs that were "deemed essential," and were therefore more likely to suffer job loss or were unable to work remotely during the pandemic. In their article, Krogstad, Hugo, and Passel (2020) illustrated that many undocumented immigrants worked in industries that were at risk for job loss during the coronavirus outbreak, because they hold positions that are difficult to perform remotely. In all, 84% of undocumented immigrant workers held such jobs in 2017, including those in the service sector (2.3 million workers) and construction sector (1.3 million workers). By comparison, 62% of U.S. citizen and legal immigrant workers held these types of jobs. Even in industries where large shares of the workforce have worked remotely, like education and health, undocumented immigrants' jobs were more likely to be in person and more difficult to telework (Krogstad et al., 2020). Immigrant families of lower socioeconomic status, therefore, were burdened with employment or child care crises during the pandemic and were likely unable to be an active part of their children's education.

Some immigrants may have also lacked formal education in English; this added a language barrier to the lack of parental presence in the home, as many recent immigrants may not have spoken the language of their child's schooling to provide any support when they were present (Brossard et al., 2020). If parents do not speak the language of instruction, it is difficult or uncomfortable for them to assist with homework or otherwise engage in their child's schooling (Goodall & Vorhaus, 2010). This once again reinforced the need for the older siblings, who were generally more fluent in the English language, to be the teacher and the helper when it came to younger students completing assignments (Wikle et al., 2018).

In addition, there were more educational disruptions for children of immigrant families rather than for those from non-immigrant families. Some immigrant families experienced difficulties when it came to moving conditions, varying school sites, family separation, and overall mental health. For example, some immigrant families opted to return to their native countries during the pandemic. Families found it was more cost-effective to support their families while they lived abroad while avoiding the cost of living in more expensive cities (Mencutek, 2021). A recent study on migration during pandemics reported that immigrants working below their qualifications in the countries to which they immigrated, were more likely to return to their native countries, as ties to homeland and economic security played critical roles in immigrants' decisions to return to their respective home countries (Mencutek, 2021).

Under those conditions, younger DLLs were not only losing the opportunity for English language immersion that is so critical in language development (U.S. Department of Health & Human Services, 2022), but were also likely dealing with logistical issues such as internet connectivity and different time zones.

In addition to the difficulties of online learning, young children from families relocating during the pandemic had the added burden of being apart from their loved ones. In many cases, younger children also had to deal with separation from their families due to deportation, work visas expiring related to job loss, or forced relocation due to other personal economic or social concerns, (Mencutek, 2021). On the other hand, travel restrictions had negative results for immigrant families. Because of travel restrictions, migrants or even visiting family members were unable to return to their native countries; this led to poorer health outcomes as more crowded households had a higher chance for disease spreading (Mobarak & Khan, 2021).

Furthermore, immigrant families fared poorer health outcomes since many immigrants held jobs deemed "essential," and those going to work and returning home were more likely to spread disease in potentially cramped conditions (Krogstad et al., 2020). Younger students may have already struggled immensely with online learning with these types of living conditions, as the lack of support with completing assignments or resolving internet connectivity issues when the adults in the household were ill led to more learning disruptions.

All the aforementioned factors for immigrant families led to a negative impact on young children's mental health both during the pandemic and in the subsequent years upon their return to typical in-person elementary education. Whereas non-immigrant children in early childhood education only had to handle the transition between virtual back to in-person education, children of immigrant families (both those that had to relocate and those confined to their homes) had to come to terms with crucial years of English language learning loss and the trauma of separation (Evans et al., 2016). Thus, the achievement gaps between DLLs and English native speakers were more pronounced with immigrant children.

The Unique Experiences of ECE Dual Language Learners

During the pandemic, a population of students that suffered the most, regardless of socioeconomic status, were DLLs. Language develops and forms in early childhood, (U.S. Department of Health & Human Services, 2022). If a young learner's linguistic traits develop mainly in a language other than English in their formative years, they can potentially struggle with English language acquisition. When early childhood students are in school, they typically grow in all languages - the language of school and those spoken at home (Evans et al., 2016). In general, not being able to understand spoken language can result in high levels of anxiety for young children, as some children who struggle to interact or have an accent may struggle socially (Kinzler et al., 2009). Because DLLs lost that consistent exposure to academic and in-person English during the pandemic's school closures, they missed valuable language-learning time in the classroom and with their peers. During the pandemic DLLs were not able to expand their four language modalities (reading, writing, listening, and speaking) as well as they would have in the school setting.

Young children sometimes often experience the social ramifications of having an accent and, therefore, feeling embarrassed or left out when it comes to communicating with their peers (Kozlowski, 2015); most students, however, overcome negative feelings because the urge to communicate and play with their peers is much stronger than any potential embarrassment they may experience (Kozlowski, 2015). Without these opportunities to engage in language learning, however, DLLs were not only missing the chance to develop language skills in the various modalities but also were not given the social openings to overcome language fears and interact with peers because they were not in school. This has led to achievement gaps for DLLs, as language acquisition needs to occur earlier to prevent gaps in reading and math in later academic years. According to a 2012 study, "DLLs who were proficient in English by kindergarten entry kept pace with native English speakers in both reading and math initially and over time; DLLs who were proficient by first grade had modest gaps in reading and math achievement compared to native English speakers that closed narrowly or persisted over time; and DLLs who were not proficient by first grade had the largest initial gaps in reading and math achievement compared to native speakers, but the gap narrowed over time in reading and grew over time in math" (Halle et al., 2012). Without the benefits of in-person learning and interaction with peers in their age group to develop both the social and academic language needed to thrive, young DLL students were inevitably forced behind academically during the pandemic.

Lessons Learned and Implications for Policy

Schools function as a critical center for societies. They offer child care and education, a reliable food source, services for DLLs, and extracurricular activities for students. When schools closed during the COVID-19 pandemic, the true gaps in society were made evident. Not only was there a disruption in education - the forced school shutdown of the pandemic further proved social disparities: people of low socioeconomic status need schools and the services they offer, whereas people of higher socioeconomic status are less likely to rely on schools to meet basic needs. While lower-income families had to struggle to financially support their children and focused heavily on putting food on the table, wealthier families had the financial and educational resources to facilitate their own means of learning for their children, through learning pods or private education (Moyer, 2020).

A beacon of light during the school closures of the pandemic was government initiatives to assist local communities in adjusting to remote learning. Many schools across the United States offered free breakfast and lunches during the pandemic, so families would still have access to free and nutritious meals despite school closures (School Nutrition Association, 2023; Zimmerman et al., 2021). This initiative was an acknowledgment from state and local governments that schools provide essential services to their respective communities in addition to education. iPads and laptops were also loaned to students during the academic year to ensure they would be able to complete assignments (Wittbold et al., 2020). This initiative also demonstrated policymakers' awareness that most students need access to devices to be part of a rapidly advancing society relying heavily on successfully using technology.

Accessibility to technology also presented schools and local governments with the opportunity to affect change. One example of a policy initiative that has had the potential to bridge was an initiative by the New York City Department of Education to recalibrate resources so that they can be accessible with just a phone (Banks, 2023). This is an example of policy initiatives for continued online learning as it allows students of all socioeconomic statuses to be able to access the same resources regardless of the type of device they can afford. Many of the technological tools developed or popularized during the pandemic have helped special populations. For example, features of the Google Suite and platforms such as ClassDojo, TalkingPoints, and Jupiter have helped teachers communicate with families of diverse linguistic backgrounds in their home language. This is especially important in early childhood, as it gives families a sense of involvement in their child's education. Another example is online writing features in Google Classrooms; DLLs can use Google's translation features or take time with writing and can get individualized feedback on Google Classroom to progress and work more effectively with the visuals that assist them in learning. The social ramifications of extra help are minimized because feedback and modified tasks can be assigned discreetly (Wullschleger et al., 2020). These technologies should continue to expand and help students and families of diverse backgrounds.

Policymakers have gained an understanding of the resources schools provide in terms of nutrition and access to reliable technology because society was forced to do without schools' resources; a valuable next step would be to collaborate with educators to provide educational resources to families as well. Policymakers should explore ways of making services or resources more accessible to parents outside of the classroom. Similarly, policies should explore ways of adequately preparing families of all socioeconomic backgrounds to take advantage of these services and resources through remote sessions and during the summer when schools are not in session.

To further implement improvements in education, UNESCO has supported parent involvement programs around the globe. These initiatives ensure that families are able to engage in their child's education regardless of education or work schedule. Specifically, the Home Instruction for Parents of Preschool Youngsters (HIPPY) program has a "focus on marginalized or disadvantaged parents or ethnic minority families" (UNESCO, 2021). The HIPPY program operates in fifteen countries, including the United States, and is facilitated in seven languages (HIPPY International, 2021). Creating more programs like this across the world, and honing in on specific minority groups within target areas that need the most support could help close achievement gaps and prepare young learners to become active agents of their own learning as they move forward through their education.

Conclusion

During the pandemic, families of lower socioeconomic status experienced more trials and tribulations than their more affluent counterparts due to the lack of ability for parents to be present and involved because of demanding work schedules, young children did not always have the opportunity to learn from their parents. Young children in families of lower socioeconomic status mostly learned either from older siblings or screens, which led to poor growth in math and reading skills (Betthäuser et al., 2023). Children of wealthier families were more likely to make academic gains because of the availability of parental involvement and resources in the home. Furthermore, immigrant children and DLLs experienced additional unique challenges. Nevertheless, some of the lessons learned during these times can prove useful in supporting young children's education from diverse backgrounds in the future.

In the 2016 Toolkit of Resources for Engaging and the Community as Partners in Education, Dean and colleagues report that "Family, school, and community have overlapping spheres of influence, and if the three spheres interact and communicate with one another, students are more likely to receive common messages about their success (Epstein, 2010)." By partnering with communities (for example, businesses, faith-based organizations, or community centers), families and schools can maximize their efforts to support student success (Epstein et al., 2002). Research shows that all students can benefit when all stakeholders work together (Dean et al., 2016). Rather than focusing on student deficits or families' cultural and socioeconomic differences, learning communities can work together to ensure that the common goals and standards for students are achieved.

Using both traditional learning and innovative online approaches will help all students master content and bridge learning gaps. The technological tools developed during the pandemic will continue to revolutionize the educational field - and can ideally become the great equalizers. Students may have varying degrees of resources in the home, but school settings can be places where all students have equal access to quality education.

References

Anders, J. (2022, December 5). *How has covid-19 affected inequalities between state and private schools?* How has COVID-19 affected inequalities between state and private schools? https://www.economicsobservatory.com/how-has-covid-19-affected-inequalities-between-state-and-private-schools.

Banks, D. (2023). *Regulation of the chancellor - New York City Department of Education.* Chancellor Banks outlines vision for transforming and building trust in NYC public schools. https://www.schools.nyc.gov/docs/default-source/default-document-library/chancellor-david-c-banks-outlines-bold-vision.

Bawalsah, J. A., & Haddad, A. H. (2020). Preferred learning styles among students with learning disabilities. *International Journal of Education, 12*(3), 119. https://doi.org/10.5296/ije.v12i3.17265.

Betthäuser, B. A., Bach-Mortensen, A. M., & Engzell, P. (2023, January 30). *A systematic review and meta-analysis of the evidence on learning during the COVID-19 pandemic.* Nature News. https://www.nature.com/articles/s41562-022-01506-4.

Blad, E. (2022, October 25). *Special education during the pandemic, in charts.* Special Education. https://www.edweek.org/teaching-learning/special-education-during-the-pandemic-in-charts/2022/10.

Bodrova, E., & Leong, D. J. (April, 2003). The importance of being playful. *Educational Leadership,* 60 (7), 50-53.

Bowles, N. (2018, October 26). The digital gap between rich and poor kids is not what we expected. https://www.nytimes.com/2018/10/26/style/digital-divide-screens-schools.html.

Bradley, K. (2023, August 2). *The socioeconomic achievement gap in the US public schools.* Ballard Brief. https://ballardbrief.byu.edu/issue-briefs/the-socioeconomic-achievement-gap-in-the-us-public-schools#:~:text=students%20enter%20high%20school%20with,behind%20their%20high%20SES%20counterparts.&text=low%20SES%20students%20are%20behind,compared%20to%20high%20SES%20students.&text=The%20success%20rate%20of%20low,lower%20than%20high%20SES%20students.

Brookings. (2010). *Immigrant Workers in the U.S. Labor Force.* New American Economy. https://www.newamericaneconomy.org/sites/all/themes/pnae/img/Immigrant_Workers_Brookings.pdf.

Brossard, M., Kamei, A., Mishra, S., Mizunoya, S., & Reuge, N. (2020, May). Parental Involvement in Children's Learning. https://www.researchgate.net/publication/342278281_Parental_Involvement_in_Children's_Learning.

Dean, C., Flores, N., Frunzi, K., Garcia, M., & Miller, K. (2016, January). *Toolkit of resources for engaging families and the community as partners in Education. part 1: Building an understanding of family and community engagement.* Institute of Education Sciences (IES) Home Page, a part of the U.S. Department of Education. https://ies.ed.gov/ncee/rel/Products/Region/pacific/Publication/3767.

Division of Information and Marketing Services. (2022, September 1). *A profile of the working poor, 2020 : BLS Reports*. U.S. Bureau of Labor Statistics. https://www.bls.gov/opub/reports/working-poor/2020/home.htm.

Evans, M., Schneider, C., Arnot, M., Fisher, L., Forbes, K., Hu, M., & Liu, Y. (2016, June). *Language development and school achievement*. Executive Summary. https://www.educ.cam.ac.uk/research/programmes/ealead/Executive_Summary.pdf.

Feifel, B., & Westheimer, Miriam. (2021). *HIPPY Around the World*. HIPPY International. https://hippy-international.org/worldwide/.

Frost, R. (2021, September 8). *Pandemic highlights disparities in high-speed internet service*. Housing Perspectives. https://www.jchs.harvard.edu/blog/pandemic-highlights-disparities-high-speed-internet-service.

Goodall, J., & Vorhaus, J. (2010). (rep.). *Review of best practice in parental engagement*. United Kingdom Department for Education. https://assets.publishing.service.gov.uk/government/uploads/system/uploads/attachment_data/file/182508/DFE-RR156.pdf.

Halle, T., Hair, E., Wandner, L., McNamara, M., & Chien, N. (2012). Predictors and outcomes of early versus later English language proficiency among English language learners. *Early Childhood Research Quarterly*, *27*(1), 1–20. https://doi.org/10.1016/j.ecresq.2011.07.004.

Hess, A. J. (2019, October 13). *People who work from home earn more than those who commute-here's why*. CNBC. https://www.cnbc.com/2019/10/13/people-who-work-from-home-earn-more-than-those-who-commuteheres-why.html

Karoly, L. (2015). *A Costly Divide: The Economic Impact of Gaps in Student Performance in Pennsylvania.* https://doi.org/10.7249/rb9872

Kinzler, K. D., Shutts, K., DeJesus, J., & Spelke, E. S. (2009). Accent trumps race in guiding children's Social Preferences. *Social Cognition, 27*(4), 623–634. https://doi.org/10.1521/soco.2009.27.4.623

Kozlowski, A. (2015). The Influence of Accents on Social Perception. *Inkblot, 4,* 12–16. https://inkblotuoft.files.wordpress.com/2015/06/alexandra1.pdf.

Lamiani, G., Borghi, L., Bonazza, F., Rebecchi, D., Lazzari, D., & Vegni, E. (2022). Adjustment Processes After the First Wave of the COVID-19 Pandemic: A Grounded Theory Study Based on Clinical Psychologists' Experience. *Secondary Psychology for Clinical Settings, 13.* https://doi.org/https://doi.org/10.3389/fpsyg.2022.854745.

Mantagas, A. (2023, April 5). *Challenges in Teaching & Learning Post-Pandemic.* Molloy University. personal. https://docs.google.com/document/d/1JJ6KWlK6fVqraxIqQUIckhVBS_G8YBX9isJOf4znwGk/edit?usp=sharing.

Masonbrink, A. R., & Hurley, E. (2020). Advocating for children during the covid-19 school closures. *Pediatrics, 146*(3). https://doi.org/10.1542/peds.2020-1440.

Mays, K., & Long, M. (2020). *The digital divide in education just got a lot wider.* Ewing Marion Kauffman Foundation. Retrieved July 5, 2023, from https://www.kauffman.org/currents/digital-divide-education-covid-19/.

McClain, C., Vogels, E. A., Perrin, A., Sechopoulos, S., & Rainie, L. (2021, September 1). *The internet and the pandemic.* Pew Research Center: Internet, Science & Tech. https://www.pewresearch.org/internet/2021/09/01/the-internet-and-the-pandemic/.

Mencutek, Z.S. (2022). Voluntary and Forced Return Migration Under a Pandemic Crisis. In: Triandafyllidou, A. (eds) *Migration and Pandemics.* IMISCOE Research Series. Springer, Cham. https://doi.org/10.1007/978-3-030-81210-2_10

Méndez, I., Jorquera Hernández, A. B., & Ruiz-Esteban, C. (2020, October 15). *Profiles of mobile phone problem use in bullying and cyberbullying among adolescents.* Frontiers in psychology. https://www.ncbi.nlm.nih.gov/pmc/articles/PMC7593657/

Miller, B. R., & Williams-Isom, A. (2021). *What COVID-19 is revealing about NYC schools: are we learning our lessons? Fordham Urban Law Journal.* 5(48), 521–545. https://ir.lawnet.fordham.edu/cgi/viewcontent.cgi?article=2833&context=ulj.

Mobarak, A. M., & Khan, M. (2021, January 21). *COVID-19 is pushing migrants back to their home countries.* openDemocracy. https://www.opendemocracy.net/en/pandemic-border/covid-19-pushing-migrants-back-their-home-countries/

Moyer, M. W. (2020, July 22). *Pods, microschools and tutors: can parents solve the education crisis on their own?* The New York Times. https://www.nytimes.com/2020/07/22/parenting/school-pods-coronavirus.html.

National Council for Special Education. (2021, June). Using visuals to support communication. https://ncse.ie/wp-content/uploads/2021/06/Using-Visuals-to-Support-Communication.pdf.

Pandey, E. (2021, January 2). *Private schools pull students away from public schools.* Axios: Economy & Business. https://www.axios.com/2021/01/02/private-schools-coronavirus-public-schools.

Quintero, D., & Hansen, M. (2022, March 9). *As we tackle school segregation, don't forget about English learner students.* Brookings Commentary. https://www.brookings.edu/articles/as-we-tackle-school-segregation-dont-forget-about-english-learner-students/#:~:text=Given%20the%20disadvantaged%20family%20backgrounds,are%20commonly%20high%2Dpoverty%20schools.

School Nutrition Association. (2023). *School meal statistics.* School Meal Statistics. https://schoolnutrition.org/about-school-meals/school-meal-statistics/.

Schultz, B. (2022, November 4). *Schools clash with parents over bans on student cellphones.* amNewYork. https://www.amny.com/education/schools-clash-with-parents-over-bans-on-student-cellphones/.

Schwab, J. F., & Lew-Williams, C. (2016). Language learning, socioeconomic status, and child-directed speech. *Wiley Interdisciplinary Reviews: Cognitive Science,* 7(4), 264–275. https://doi.org/10.1002/wcs.1393.

Shrider, E. A., Kollar, M., Chen, F., & Semega, J. (2021, September). *Current population reports: Income and Poverty in the United States: 2020.* United

States Census. https://www.census.gov/content/dam/Census/library/publications/2021/demo/p60-273.pdf?stream=top.

UNESCO. (2021, September 22). *Parental support to learning*. Parental support to learning | UNESCO IIEP Learning Portal. https://learningportal.iiep.unesco.org/en/issue-briefs/improve-learning/parental-support-to-learning.

United States Department of Health & Human Services. (2022, October 13). *Speech and language developmental milestones*. National Institute of Deafness and Other Communication Disorders. https://www.nidcd.nih.gov/health/speech-and-language#:~:text=The%20first%203%20years%20of,speech%20and%20language%20of%20others.

Vogels, E. A. (2020, September 10). *59% of U.S. parents with lower incomes say their child may face digital obstacles in schoolwork*. Pew Research Center. https://www.pewresearch.org/short-reads/2020/09/10/59-of-u-s-parents-with-lower-incomes-say-their-child-may-face-digital-obstacles-in-schoolwork/.

Wikle, J. S., Jensen, A. C., & Hoagland, A. M. (2018). Adolescent caretaking of younger siblings. *Social Science Research, 71*, 72–84. https://doi.org/10.1016/j.ssresearch.2017.12.007

Wittbold, K. A., Baugh, J. J., Yun, B. J., Raja, A. S., & White, B. A. (2020). IPad deployment for virtual evaluation in the Emergency Department during the COVID-19 pandemic. *The American Journal of Emergency Medicine, 38*(12), 2733–2734. https://doi.org/10.1016/j.ajem.2020.04.025.

Wullschleger, A., Garrote, A., Schnepel, S., Jaquiéry, L., & Moser Opitz, E. (2020). Effects of teacher feedback behavior on social acceptance in inclusive elementary classrooms: Exploring social referencing processes in a natural setting. *Contemporary Educational Psychology, 60*, 101841. https://doi.org/10.1016/j.cedpsych.2020.101841.

Zimmerman, E., Griffen, S., & Hauer, J. (2021, September 24). *COVID-19 the Family, State and Federal Policy: Lessons Learned in New England.* U.S. Department of Health & Human Services: Office of Regional Operations. https://www.acf.hhs.gov/sites/default/files/documents/oro/oro_covid_19_resources_update_1.pdf.

About the Contributing Author:

Anna Mantagas holds an MSED in TESOL (Teaching English to Speakers of Other Languages), Advanced Certification in Teaching Students with Disabilities, and is currently completing an MA in School District Leadership. She teaches English Language Learners, Students with Disabilities, and Acting in New York City Public Schools. She also works as an Adjunct Faculty at Pace University's School of Education. Her mission is to bring the joys of reading and language to English Language Learners and Students with Disabilities through Theatre Arts. She splits her time between teaching in New York and spending time in her native Cyprus. She lives in Astoria, Queens with her husband and two children.

Chapter 6
COVID-19 and the Experiences of Young Children with Disabilities

Jennifer Pankowski, Ruth Guirguis, and Raquel Plotka

The United States educates about seven million students with disabilities ages 3-21 annually in public school systems. Even though this number represents approximately 15% of the national population, the needs of the individuals, their families, educators, service providers, and administrators tasked with supporting these children were not met during the COVID-19 crisis when most schools abruptly shut down face to face instruction. Children with disabilities were disproportionately negatively impacted during this time (National Center for Education Statistics, 2023).

The impact of the COVID-19 pandemic on education has forced a deep look into both the historical significance and subsequent implementation of special education legislation during the forced school shutdowns and lack of access for children. This chapter presents a literature review coupled with extensive examination of public data from local, national, and international organizations during and after the COVID-19 pandemic, exposing several shortcomings, risks, and inequalities in the education of students with disabilities within the United States. The pandemic not only revealed the vulnerabilities within the special education system, but it opened the ongoing dialogue on critical issues about the future of special education in a post-pandemic world.

Prior to COVID-19, the U.S. had legislation protecting all children from birth to age 21 with disabilities for many years; during the pandemic, however, many educational organizations failed to protect students with disabilities. These students received substandard education, which contributed to the well-documented rise in the number of impartial hearings with claims regarding these experiences (New York State Department of Education, 2023). Impartial hearings focus on protecting due process rights for students with disabilities. In recent years, impartial hearings have frequently cited complaints addressing the inability of schools to provide consistent and appropriate access to related services, as well as improper class ratios (a national concern even before the COVID-19 pandemic). The lack of both access and resources due to the COVID-19 pandemic has only proven to exacerbate these ongoing concerns present before the pandemic. Perhaps one of the most severely impacted groups during this time is early childhood education (ECE) students who rely on proper services for early intervention (EI) and early identification of needs. Without proper resources for identification, and early assessment screenings, young students with disabilities were often left without the services and support they needed during the pandemic closures and into the months and years that followed.

History of Special Education and Equal Access

Before developing a system of accountability in special education, the United States was party to numerous human rights violations relating to students and individuals with disabilities. One example of such a violation was the Willowbrook State School. Willowbrook was a New York State-supported institution (1947-1988) for children with intellectual disabilities. While the school was designed for 4,000 student residents, from 1965 until its forced closure in 1988, it had a population of more than 6,000 residents. The conditions, medical practices, and experiments on children were questioned as early as 1972 after an expose that led to the closure in 1988 (Bursztyn, 2006). While action was eventually taken to address these human rights violations, it took over a decade for accountability to be taken for the mistreatment of these children. Just as society continues to use the atrocities of Willowbrook State School to discuss its impact on special education decades after its closure, it is likely that the impacts of COVID-19 on all students, particularly those with disabilities, will be discussed for decades to come to avoid similar inequities again.

The Individuals with Disabilities Education Act (IDEA) passed into federal law in 1975, over two hundred years after the United States was established in 1776. Before the establishment of legislation to ensure equal educational opportunities for special education, millions of children were denied adequate schooling. Also, during that time, raising, supporting, and educating these children fell almost exclusively on families unless the child was placed into a care facility or publicly run institution. The rights of people with disabilities did not have a specific notation in federal legislation until the passage of the Rehabilitation Act (1973); more specifically, Section 504 of the Rehabilitation Act mandates nondiscrimination for people with disabilities in educational programs if those programs receive federal funding. This act was followed by the Education for All Handicapped Children Act (1975), which guarantees a free and appropriate public education (FAPE) for every child with a disability in the United States. These legislations have changed how students with disabilities are educated in the United States by mandating that disabilities have an identification and treatment process so that families of children with disabilities are able to exercise their right to due process.

Part B of the IDEA focuses on special education services for preschoolers ages 3-5 with disabilities and their families. Preschoolers can receive services after an evaluation has transpired. An Individualized Education Plan (IEP) is developed after the evaluation, and the IEP outlines the needs of the child and their families and a plan for interventions. Part C of the IDEA focuses on early intervention services for infants and toddlers with disabilities and delays and resources for their families. This critical section provides support and services to promote the development and well-being of young children with disabilities and to support their families in supporting their children. Hence, young children from birth until age three can receive services after an evaluation has transpired. An Individualized Family Service Plan (IFSP) is developed after the evaluation process; it outlines the needs of the child and their families and a plan for interventions. According to this section of the law, young learners should receive support services in their natural environments, such as within their ECE classrooms or their homes.

The COVID-19 pandemic has raised many concerns for families and educators that were once thought to be addressed historically with federal legislation. Decades after the implementation of Parts B and C of the IDEA, families were again left with the burden of raising, supporting, and educating their young children.

The term "student with disabilities" can have several definitions as students with disabilities participate in a range of educational settings, such as general education classes with additional support, inclusive co-teaching, self-contained classrooms, as well as related service push-ins and pull-outs. Additionally, some students use adaptive technology to participate in residential programs. The present chapter has focused on ECE students who attend public and private preschools that receive support services and have IEPs or IFSPs.

The Impacts of COVID-19 on Young Children with Disabilities

Although students have returned to "pre-pandemic" status once again and in-person class structures have resumed, the impacts from COVID-19 are far from resolved. Students with disabilities, particularly those from historically marginalized subgroups, have continued to experience the detrimental effects of the COVID-19 pandemic. As more studies continue to focus on the long-term impacts of the pandemic, findings point to lack of access to services, ineffective remote instruction, and the critical impact social distancing had on skill development; all of these were significant contributors as to why students with disabilities are now presenting with delays and disabilities in several areas of development such as language and social and emotional development, in addition to their previous diagnoses (Pattnaik et al, 2022; UNESCO for Institute for Information Technologies in Education, 2021; Lipkin & Crepeau-Hobson, 2022).

For young children, these inequities have had lasting impacts. The crisis left students needing access to proven interventions that are most effective when offered consistently at an early age. In the fall of 2020, the Centers for Disease Control and Prevention (2020) conducted a rapid assessment for young children from birth to age five. COVID-19 pandemic had an impact on the early identification of children with developmental delays and disabilities. The assessment has highlighted needs, barriers, and gaps in for early recognition and treatment of developmental delay and disability among children from birth to age five during the COVID-19 pandemic.

These barriers and gaps have resulted in deficits for children in the areas of cognitive development and academic skills, language development, social and emotional development and self-regulated behaviors. In addition, these gaps had negative effects on educators, families, and service providers. The following sections describe several effects of COVID-19 for children with delays or disabilities.

Effects on Cognitive Development and Academic Success

Cognitive development is supported by the environmental conditions present during early development. The quality of preschools and qualified ECE teachers can promote academic gains. During the pandemic, school closures and a lack of skilled professionals to teach young learners hindered growth. Caregivers who were not educators were responsible for a significant part of student learning (Timmons et al., 2021). Consequently, lessons through online platforms did not have the same quality of instruction as pre-COVID lessons (Timmons et al., 2021). As a result, there was a lack of engagement in young children that required additional caregiver support, making it challenging for adults to work and provide instruction simultaneously.

The U.S. Department of Education (2021) highlighted that widespread barriers caused by lack of access to adequate education during the pandemic, negatively affected academic growth by widening pre-existing disparities in core subjects like math and reading. While the short and long-term impacts on cognitive development are still unknown, there is limited information suggesting several negative impacts. For example, children's engagement and attention significantly decreased during online instruction, impacting their learning (Timmons et al., 2021).

Early literacy and math skill development are at the cornerstone of ECE. ECE plays a critical role in identifying skill deficits early and implementing early interventions to support young children with disabilities. ECE is often the first academic setting for children and where data collected by teachers and related service providers becomes an important foundation for future educational services. During the COVID-19 pandemic, resources needed to support ECE were limited and non-existent, and, as such, left lasting impacts on academic success for many young children with disabilities.

The effects of COVID-19 on academics in ECE are especially significant when it comes to language and literacy development. As Timmons et al. (2021) noted, the early primary grades are essential for the acquisition of foundational language and literacy; this is because language and literacy skills develop as children learn to communicate both verbally and non-verbally. ECE settings are an opportunity to make language meaningful through communication. Thus, ECE teachers continuously assess the literacy and language skills of ECE students on an ongoing basis to ensure they are meeting the individual learning goals of their students. Learning in ECE is often fostered through teacher-guided play-based activities, where students can be exposed to new vocabulary and narrative skills. Similarly, numeracy skills are typically acquired through play-based activities such as creating patterns, sorting items, and estimating (Ginsberg, 2006). With the sudden shift to remote instruction, teachers and students lost the ability to engage in this type of meaningful play. Very young children were faced with learning critical academic skills, such as language and literacy, using methods not designed for young children.

When classrooms across the globe pivoted to remote instruction, teachers were tasked with the seemingly impossible task of providing instruction in a new remote classroom environment for special education teachers and paraprofessionals who rely on one-on-one individual instruction and opportunities to support students academically with verbal, gestural, and other prompting to help young children communicate. Having to pivot to remote instruction limited the opportunities for certain types of teaching such as one-on-one, hand-over-hand support, physical prompting, and "circulating a room." Special educators relied on private remote meetings for only part of the day with each child when possible or navigating group instruction to their best capacity. Teaching in the siloed remote environment also meant special education teachers and paraprofessionals could not effectively collaborate with related service providers to link support to academic instruction, and there was no way to ensure services were being provided. As much as 46% of students living in urban areas with disabilities received only part of the interventions impacting their cognitive and academic development (Lee & Luellen, 2020).

Effects on Social and Emotional Development

Initial research suggests that the trauma associated with the COVID-19 pandemic and the changes in and lack of community services and support for students with disabilities might have triggered or exacerbated pre-existing vulnerabilities, thus further widening the gap in children's social skills and ability to display appropriate behaviors (Marazziti et al., 2020).

Due to the characteristics associated with many students supported by special education, a hallmark strategy of educating students with disabilities is the focus on consistency and structured routine. The school shutdowns during the COVID-19 pandemic ended that for students, and due to the abrupt nature of both the pandemic and the widespread school closings, there was no time to prepare students to transition into a remote environment. This meant students were often left feeling higher levels of anxiety and inability to pivot into a new learning environment. This also left parents and caregivers solely tasked with the mental and, at times physical, responsibility of supporting their child(ren) emotionally, physically, and academically. Jobs typically filled by multiple professionals were now the burden of individual families who are not typically skilled in providing these types of support in an academic setting.

Loss of routine and structure exacerbated challenging behaviors, which made learning near impossible. In addition, the lack of support for teachers and families in how to deal with those behaviors has further contributed to the devastating impacts of the COVID-19 pandemic on children's social and emotional development. For many children, even the return to a familiar schedule was not enough to counteract the detrimental effects of losing them to begin with. Thus, many students have suffered behavioral regression that has forced them to re-learn self-coping and regulating strategies to function in the classroom environment.

Ma et al. (2020) determined that COVID-19 impacted children's behaviors, sleep, communication, and diet. Over one-third of the students exhibited problem behaviors, such as hyperactivity, with a significant correlation between affect and behavior (Ma et al., 2020). As a result of this lack of routine, parents were forced to develop informal coping measures to address problem behaviors. The use of a structured routine is a crucial component of special education; however, Mete Yesil et al. (2022) found that 76.5% of children's daily routines worsened, with the median screen time increasing from 1 to 3 hours.

Both aforementioned studies highlighted that, while the lockdown and school closings did allow families to spend more time together, replicating the extensive support found in the special education classroom to accommodate students with disabilities proved a difficult task for parents and caregivers. Students experienced regression in their ability to maintain their routines and therefore socio-emotional development suffered (Ma et al., 2020; Mete Yesil et al., 2022). Without the extensive resources needed to recreate the classroom environment at home, parents were forced to create informal strategies and coping mechanisms to help their child(ren) survive the daily stress and anxiety.

Lack of social connection, virtual learning, and change management hinder the positive development of young children's stress levels (Lipkin & Crepeau-Hobson, 2022). Additionally, students' sensory regulation was negatively impacted as they were constantly in front of a computer rather than moving around in a classroom with peer interactions (Lipkin & Crepeau-Hobson, 2022). As a result, children were observed to be disengaged and to have more behavioral outbursts (Lipkin & Crepeau-Hobson, 2022).

This regression in behaviors and self-regulatory skills has been reflected in student suspension rates when schools reopened. For example, in large cities such as New York City, student suspension rates rose a staggering 27% in the 2021 academic year following the return to school (Zimmerman, 2023). The New York City statistics following a May 2022 National Center for Education Statistics survey that found more than 80% of public schools had noticed delayed behavioral and socio-emotional development in students amid the pandemic. Educators also reported smaller, but still notable, increases in observed bullying and violence (Shen-Berro, 2023).

COVID-19 and ECE Early Intervention Services and Supports

During the move to remote instruction, some services students desperately needed were not conducive to a remote environment, particularly Physical Therapy (PT) and Occupational Therapy (OT), which require physical support. In many cases, related services and therapies that typically require hands-on, face-to-face interaction or specialized equipment – like occupational or physical therapy – had to be provided remotely, with limited effectiveness (United States Department of Education, 2021). Related service providers shifted to remote instruction, which left these professionals with a compromised situation that did not permit them to provide full academic support for students with disabilities. This deficit continued even when in-person instruction resumed, as the mandates for social distancing did not support students who require physical prompting and support, whether it be learning how to navigate stairs safely, hold a pencil, or learn essential Adaptive Daily Living Skills (ADLs) such as manipulating buttons and zippers for dressing and toileting. Thus, these necessary services could not be provided in an academic environment of social distancing.

Similarly, to the extent that COVID-19 added risks for professionals in the medical community, special education teachers and students were required to take on this additional burden for proper special education services to be delivered. As a result, staff and teachers were forced to decide between the risk to their own health and providing necessary support. For medically fragile students, families had to wrestle with the choice between prioritizing health or education (Nelson, 2020).

Finally, services for children from birth to three are supposed to take place in the home environment. This resulted in an additional challenge exacerbated by the COVID-19 pandemic, which demonstrated the inequities in marginalized communities. Access to these resources became even more limited and several young learners of lower socioeconomic status (SES) did not have the space or resources in the home to receive these support services.

COVID-19 Effects on ECE Families and Caregivers

During the COVID pandemic, parents and caregivers were left to find related services and child care. This resulted in a financial drain for private services, and for many children this resulted in no services at all. The impact on families of students with disabilities due of school closures was more pronounced than for other families, as simply having children sit in front of a computer for instruction or allowing them screen time so caregivers can work does not work for this group. Families were then left in a particularly difficult and lonely situation during the lockdown and remote instruction. For many, the regression of skills during this time has still not rebounded to a pre-pandemic level for their children with disabilities, even though most students have returned to in-person instruction.

Findings suggest that the rapid changes in social life associated with restrictions put in place to prevent the spread of the COVID-19 virus resulted in increased anxiety in families of children with disabilities and negatively impacted the mood and behaviors of both children and their families (Asbury et al., 2021; Gayatri & Irawaty, 2021). As previously mentioned, routine and structure are critical components of the special education classroom setting, and when these routines are disrupted, so is the ability to learn socially, emotionally, and academically. When classrooms were closed, parents were focused on creating the missing routines for their children, and they struggled through a trial-and-error process to find what worked and what did not. Parents had to encourage their children to engage with virtual education initially and in-person education that looks much different than before COVID-19. This additional burden left parents not just as caregivers but also teachers, lunch monitors, school nurses, and related service providers - all of this on top of tending to their jobs, roles, and other responsibilities. This had direct and indirect impacts on the family's quality of life as it relates to the perceived social support, parent self-efficacy, and psychological resilience of parents (Rakap et al., 2022).

Parents of children with disabilities experienced higher levels of stress and concern during the lockdown and additional pressure to reconcile their caregiving role with their paid employment, especially when compared to parents of children without disabilities (Hochman et al., 2022). Without a school's resources, the interventions designed help ensure an equal educational opportunity developed and implemented by the child's school team of particular support providers; the burden falls squarely on the families (Lipkin & Crepeau-Hobson, 2022). For many parents, the pressures of caring for their children with disabilities resulted in an inability to continue to work, which put additional financial strains on the family.

Lessons Learned

Reflection is critical in ensuring lessons have been learned during challenging times. What society has learned about education, both generally and specifically, from the COVID-19 pandemic is that future preparation and understanding of inequities are key in preventing the type of lost learning that has occurred during this period. Although the full extent of the impacts on young ECE students with disabilities is not yet fully known, a review of the existing information has highlighted several deficits and pathways for future change. Several lessons were learned during this trial-and-error period that can help guide future practice. The following section discusses implications for supporting engagement and instruction, children's social and emotional development, communication with families, the various referral processes, and policy considerations.

Lessons for Engagement and Instruction

The COVID-19 unearthed systemic issues that need to be addressed moving forward by examining and quantifying the impacts of missed instruction and related services for students with disabilities. ECE educators need more professional development opportunities that support teaching through online platforms. While in-person education is critical for young students, some aspects of special education can continue to be implemented online. For example, online teacher and family meetings increased the support that families gave young students at home. The flexibility of timing in educators having virtual learning support sessions increased due to COVID-19. Teachers can discuss support strategies and materials to be used at home with students in a time and space that works for caregivers. Thus, increasing teacher accessibility online can be a positive instruction component.

Continued support of ECE educators with digital literacy and computational thinking skills will be essential, as society enters a more technological setting. While ECE is an in-person profession, with the COVID-19 pandemic, the need for computational thinking and digital skills has become more prevalent in education and among young children (Jain et al., 2021). As technology is implemented in the classroom, teachers need to be able to identify platforms that measure and teach what is intended and assess if these platforms are developmentally appropriate. Technology as an additional support in the classroom, not as the primary form of learning, can improve young children's academic outcomes if factors such as student preference towards utilizing technology exist and if the ECE classroom teacher is familiar with the technology and can actively participate (Paul et al., 2023). Hence, ongoing technological professional development for teachers is needed.

Lesson in Supporting Social-Emotional Development

Students who typically receive extensive support and services in the classroom regressed in their observable social and emotional skills during the COVID-19 lockdown (Morando-Rhim & Ekin, 2021). While schools tried to prioritize children with disabilities to be back in the classroom, many remained online. Additionally, parameters for providing services online were not set, influencing the decline of social and emotional skills in ECE (Morando-Rhim & Ekin, 2021).

A key lesson learned during the COVID-19 lockdown was the central role of play in supporting social and emotional skills. "Play sets the foundation for the development of critical social and emotional knowledge and skills. Through play, children learn to forge connections with others and to share, negotiate, and resolve conflicts, as well as learn self-advocacy skills. Play also teaches children leadership as well as group skills" (UNICEF 2020, p. 10). Additionally, play-based learning allows young students to cooperate with their peers and display socially appropriate behavior (Egin et al., 2021). Specifically, play allows young students to develop language and positive social skills. In ECE play, play-based activities allow practitioners to observe, scaffold learning, while working on the IEP and IFSP goals.

Many ECE educators included several interactive activities during online instruction. For example, teachers incorporated story time online with props and interactive materials that were engaging for young learners during online instruction. Similarly, teachers organized scavenger hunts and other activities for children to connect their home experiences with the online audience. Emotional check-ins were essential during the lockdown. ECE teachers have had children identify their feelings by using charts or visuals. This allowed young learners to express their feelings and have teachers support them through individualized activities. Music instruction has also been revealed to positively connect with social and emotional learning (Xia & Li, 2022), as music instruction and musical activities reduce negative emotions and inappropriate behaviors (Xia & Li, 2022).

Another lesson learned was the effectiveness of educators scheduling virtual individual meetings with young students and their families. This created a one-on-one relationship among students, teachers, and families to support better children's well-being (Vaillacort et al., 2021), intentionally including developmentally appropriate social and emotional books, activities, and lessons. Nevertheless, the crisis highlighted the need for more professional development for ECE educators in teaching and supporting social and emotional skills in an online platform.

Lessons for the Referrals Process

Referrals and identification rates are essential in understanding and proactively addressing notable shifts in student needs. The lack of in-person services limits the early identification of young students with disabilities due to a lack of access to evidence-based tools for assessment.

While a lack of data is one lesson worth learning from, it is also essential that the practices and strategies identified during the COVID-19 be closely evaluated to determine their future use. Morando-Rhim & Ekin (2021) recommend focusing on, documenting, and validating emerging innovative approaches, such as the use of small-group learning hubs, remote instruction and teletherapy, virtual IFSP or IEP meetings, and strategies to boost parent engagement to determine their effectiveness for students with disabilities and potential to be implemented over the long term. These online platforms can make family engagement and discussions more feasible. Similarly, video observations can support the referral process and are fundamental in recommending interventions for young children. With the ease that referrals and interventions can be conducted online, ECE programs need to establish systems to identify the rate of referrals and to understand and proactively address notable shifts from pre-pandemic data. This process would require programs to collectively implement a system to collect and analyze referral data to identify rate shifts and available resources.

Policy Implications

Local Educational Agencies (LEAs) need to develop and implement plans to address the impacts of the COVID-19 pandemic on students and educators through new and existing funding streams. It is specifically important to highlight the role of special education services and the need for evidence-based learning recovery strategies and interventions to meet student needs related to COVID-19; these should respond to students' social, emotional, and academic needs and the use of individualized approaches to provide specialized instruction and related services should be consistent with students' IFSPs or IEPs. Additionally, training educators and implementing trauma-informed practices in all ECE programs can help determine how to support the academic, social, and emotional learning needs of students with disabilities during COVID-19 (Morando-Rhim & Ekin, 2021).

Conclusion

Like many watershed events in the history of education, the COVID-19 pandemic and its subsequent impacts on the education of students with disabilities will continue to impact the future of education for many years. While on the surface the impact may have appeared contained to the individual students who are served by special education and related services, it is evident through the review of the literature that the stakeholders involved are far more extensive.

Like the lessons learned from previous impacts on the education of students with disabilities, both manmade and naturally occurring, the current lessons will help improve student support in the long term. Individual reading and math scores are not the only areas of academic success that saw a direct hit due to the COVID-19 pandemic. Fortunately, not all lessons will be placed on a shelf for future "in case of emergency" situations. Many lessons relate to bridging pre-existing gaps in access that have impacted students with disabilities for many decades. Additionally, the necessity of technology highlighted that increased use of technology for children early on could help support their access to the curriculum. For many students, this shift to remote instruction presented an opportunity to find effective strategies for academic and socio-emotional growth. Data (Ma et al., 2020; Mete Yesil et al., 2022) highlighted that the COVID-19 pandemic allowed for more family time. Mete et al. (2020) noted some positive effects on the quality of family relationships, such as one-on-one time duration with the mother and father increased (73.5% and 66.7%), reading books (40.6%), and playtime (17.2%). An increase in quality time for these areas will likely prove especially impactful for young children as ECE has evidenced that this is a critical time for development (Timmons, 2020).

References

Americans With Disabilities Act of 1990, 42 U.S.C. § 12101 *et seq.* (2018). https://www.govinfo.gov/content/pkg/USCODE-2018-title42/pdf/ USCODE-2018-title42-chap126.pdf

Asbury, K., Fox, L., Deniz, E., Code, A. & Toseeb, U. (2021). How is COVID-19 affecting the mental health of children with special educational needs and disabilities and their families? *Journal of Autism and Developmental Disorders*, *51*, 1772-1780. doi:10.1007/s10803-020-04577-2

Centers for Disease Control and Prevention (2020). *Impact of the COVID-19 Pandemic on Early Identification of Developmental Delays and Disabilities and Opportunities for Improvement*. Center for Disease Control and Prevention. https://www.cdc.gov/ncbddd/actearly/pdf

Education For All Handicapped Children Act, Public Law 142, U.S. Statutes at Large 89 (1975): 773-796.

Gayatri, M., & Irawaty, D. K. (2022). Family Resilience during COVID-19 Pandemic: A Literature Review. *Family journal (Alexandria, Va.)*, *30*(2), 132–138. https://doi.org/10.1177/10664807211023875

Ginsberg, H. P. (2006). Mathematical play and playful mathematics: A guide for early education. N D. Singer, R. M. Golinkof, & HirshPasek (Eds.), Play = learning: How play motivates and enhances children's cognitive and social-emotional growth (pp. 145–165). Oxford, EN: Oxford University Press. doi:https://doi.org/10.1093/ acprof:oso/9780195304381.003.0008

Hochman, Y., Shpigelman C.N., & Holler, R.S. (2022). "Together in a pressure cooker": Parenting children with disabilities during the COVID-19 lockdown. *Disabilities Health Journal*, *15*(3):101273. doi: 10.1016/j.dhjo.2022.101273.

Individuals with Disabilities Education Act, 20 U.S.C. § 1400 (2004)

Jain, S., Lall, M., & Singh, A. (2021). Teachers' Voices on the Impact of COVID-19 on School Education: Are ed-tech companies really the panacea? *Contemporary Education Dialogue*, *18*(1), 58–89. https://doi.org/10.1177/0973184920976433

Jalongo, M. R. (2021). The effects of covid-19 on Early Childhood Education and care: Research and resources for children, families, teachers, and teacher educators. *Early Childhood Education Journal, 49*(5), 763–774. https://doi.org/10.1007/s10643-021-01208-y

Lee, H., & Luellen, J.L. (2020) Long-term head start impacts on cognitive outcomes for children with disabilities, *Families in Society: The Journal of Contemporary Social Services, 102* (1), https://doi.org/10.1177/1044389420926131

Lipkin, M. & Crepeau-Hobson, F. (2022). The impact of the COVID-19 school closures on families with children with disabilities: A qualitative analysis, *Psychology in the Schools*, 60, 1544-1559.https://doi.org/10.1002/pits.22706

Ma, M., Wang, X., Qi, P., and Wang, T. (2022). Affect, behaviors of children with intellectual disabilities and parents' coping strategies during the COVID-19 pandemic. *Frontiers in Psychiatry, 13*, doi.org/10.3389/fpsyt.2022.822908

Marazziti, D., Pozza, A., Di Giuseppe, M., & Conversano, C. (2020). The psychosocial impact of COVID-19 pandemic in Italy: A lesson for mental health prevention in the first severely hit European country. *Psychological Trauma: Theory, Research, Practice, and Policy, 12*(5), 531–533. https://doi.org/10.1037/tra0000687

Mete Yesil A, Sencan B, Omercioglu E, & Ozmert E.N., (2022) The Impact of the COVID-19 Pandemic on Children with Special Needs: A Descriptive Study. *Clinical Pediatrics, 61*(2):141-149. doi:10.1177/00099228211050223

Morando-Rhim L., Ekin S. (2021). How has the pandemic affected students with disabilities? A review of the evidence to date. *Center for Reinventing Public Education, University of Wisconsin-Madison.* https://www.crpe.org/sites/default/files/final_swd_report_2021.pdf

New York State Department of Education, (2023). *Impartial Hearing Reporting System*. New York State Department of Education. https://www.nysed.gov/special-education/impartial-hearing-reporting-system

Pattnaik J, Nath N, & Nath S. (2022). Challenges to remote instruction during the pandemic: A Qualitative study with primary grade teachers in India. *Early Child Education Journal*. doi: 10.1007/s10643-022-01331-4.

Paul, C.D., Hansen, S.G., Marelle, C. *et al.* Incorporating Technology into Instruction in Early Childhood Classrooms: a Systematic Review. *Adv*

Neurodev Disord 7, 380–391 (2023). https://doi.org/10.1007/s41252-023-00316-7

Rakap, S., Vurak-Betik, Kalkan, S., Karnas, M., Ibrahim Sari, H., & Bayrakdar, U. (2022)., The hidden (overlooked) impact of living through a pandemic: How parents of children with disabilities fared during COVID-19, *Frontiers in Education, 28(*7). https://doi.org/10.3389/feduc.2022.827230

Suriano, C. (2021). The State Education Department of The University of New York, https://www.p12.nysed.gov/specialed/publications

Timmons, K., Cooper, A., Bozek, E. *et al.* (2021). The impacts of COVID-19 on early Childhood education: Capturing the unique challenges associated with remote teaching and learning in K-2. *Early Childhood Educ Journal, 49:* 887–901. https://doi.org/10.1007/s10643-021-01207-z

UNESCO for Institute for Information Technologies in Education, (2021). Policy Brief: Understanding the impact of COVID-19 on the education of persons with disabilities: Challenges and opportunities of distance education https://unesdoc.unesco.org/ark:/48223/pf0000378404

U.S. Department of Education, Office for Civil Rights, Free Appropriate Public Education for Students With Disabilities: Requirements Under Section 504 of the Rehabilitation Act of 1973, Washington, D.C., 2010.

U.S. Department of Education. (2021). Education in a pandemic: The disparate impacts of COVID-19 on America's students, *Office of Civil Rights.* https://www2.ed.gov/about/offices/list/ocr/docs/20210608-impacts-of-covid19.pdf

Vaillancourt, T., Brittain, H., Bennett, L., Arnocky, S., McDougall, P., Hymel, S., Short, K., Sunderani, S., Scott, C., Mackenzie, M., & Cunningham, L. (2010). Places to avoid: Population-based study of student reports of unsafe and high bullying areas at school. *Canadian Journal of School Psychology*, 25(1), 40–54. https://doi.org/10.1177/0829573509358686

Washington, DC: National Center for Education Statistics (2023). Preprimary, elementary, and secondary education: Elementary and secondary enrollment, Retrieved from the Library of Congress, https://nces.ed.gov/programs/coe/pdf/2023/cgg_508.pdf

Xia, T., & Li, Z. (2022). Behavioral training of high-functioning autistic children by music education of occupational therapy. Occupational Therapy International, 2022, 1–10. https://doi.org/10.1155/2022/6040457

About the Contributing Author:

Jennifer Pankowski, Ed.D. is an Associate Professor of Special Education and the Director for Alternative Certification Programs at Pace University. She received her Ed.D in Curriculum and Instruction from Long Island University in 2013. Her research interests focus on students with disabilities, in particular the field of autism, and neurodiversity, teacher preparation, family engagement and the use of technology. Dr. Pankowski also serves as the primary U.S. researcher for the Kinems software company (Athens, Greece) and serves on the New York State Commissioner's Advisory Panel for Special Education.

Chapter 7
The Experiences of Home-Based Child Care Centers During COVID-19

Annette Pic and Myae Han

Home-based child care (HBCC) is one of two primary child care and early education (CCEE) programs in the United States. Center-based care (CBC) is the second major type of child care. Home-based child care is care provided by a non-relative in a residential setting; center-based care is public or private group care provided outside of a residential setting. Home-based child care can also include unlicensed or unlisted care (National Survey of Early Care and Education [NSECE] Project Team, 2016) that is unpaid and provided by a relative, friend, or neighbor. In this chapter, the terms HBCC, FCC, and family day homes are used interchangeably to refer to listed (licensed, regulated, license-exempt, or registered [NSECE Project Team, 2016]) and paid child care programs provided in the educator's home.

The unprecedented COVID-19 pandemic upended the child care industry as it did with a vast range of industries globally. As a whole, CCEE programs that continued to operate during the COVID pandemic faced multiple challenges, such as decreased enrollment, reduced income, higher operating costs, and psychosocial stress (Crawford et al., 2021; Kim et al., 2022; Pattnaik & Lopez, 2023). Notably, recent research suggests that HBCC programs were disproportionately impacted by the pandemic (Kim et al., 2022).

Family Preference and Use of Home-Based Child Care

In 2019, almost 60% of children birth to age 5 participated in a nonparental care arrangement (Cui & Natzke, 2021). This includes almost 6.4 million children from birth to age 5 participating in home-based child care (Datta et al., 2021). Analysis of 2012 NSECE data found that 30% of infants and toddlers participated in home-based child care compared to 12% of center-based participation (Paschall, 2019). These estimates include home-based programs that are listed and unlisted. Only three states do not have mandatory licensing requirements for any home-based providers and, currently, 44 states and the District of Columbia require HBCC licensure and the other states include HBCC in their definition of the group care home (National Center on Early Childhood Quality Assurance [NCEQA], 2020a).

Families differ in their need for non-parental care based on family and child characteristics such as employment, number of children in the home, child age, ethnicity and race, and family income (Chaudry et al., 2010; Forry et al, 2014; Weber, 2011). National estimates suggest that just under a million U.S. children attend listed HBCC arrangements (NCEQA, 2020a). Many families choose home-based care to meet their family's needs. Families select HBCCs for reasons such as affordability, location, continuity of care, scheduling flexibility, non-traditional hours, small group setting, mixed age groups, home-like setting, and cultural expectations (Banghart, 2022; Chaudry et al., 2010; Ferreira van Leer & Coley, 2023; Hill, 2021; Schilder, 2021). In fact, many families prefer FCC for their children from birth to 6 months and rank HBCC higher than CBC in terms of nurturing, affordability, and flexibility (NSECE Project Team, 2014). NSECE data reported that listed home-based care offered more flexibility in non-standard (evening and weekend) hours of care (NSECE Project Team, 2015). Home-based child care programs also offer families continuity in care for children; care for their child by the same caregiver for several years allows providers and children and their families to develop long-lasting and meaningful relationships (Theilheimer, 2010).

Government-Issued Pandemic Mandates and Stay-at-Home Orders

A state agency report conducted between April 30 and June 16, 2020, by the U.S. Department of Health and Human Services (DHSS), Office of Inspector General reported that 63% of CBC and 27% of HBCC (listed) closed during the COVID-19 pandemic. Forty-four states and the District of Columbia issued stay-at-home or shelter-in-place orders or directives designed to slow or minimize the spread of COVID-19 (DHSS, 2020). During this period, 33 states allowed ECE educators to remain open, while 17 states and the District of Columbia only allowed ECE educators to care for children of essential workers (DHSS, 2020). The state of Rhode Island closed all CCEE programs with the exception of one program that operates on a hospital campus (DHSS, 2020). These changes required that most United States education programs close or move to virtual learning (Ali et al., 2021). Further, states issued new mandates and recommendations to ensure the health and safety of child care employees, children, and families. Mandates and required program changes included suspending the use of sensory play materials, changing drop off/pick up location to minimize in-person contact, increasing cleaning and screening processes (e.g., temperature checks, health history form), reducing the number of children in their care among other recommendations (State of Delaware, 2020), strictly limiting close person-to-person contact such as hugging and games that involved touching and recommending the cancelation or modification of activities that brought children into close or direct contact (New Jersey Department of Children and Families, 2020). Child care and early education providers who chose to continue to operate in-person care did so without much support or resources (Weiland et al., 2021).

Current Study

The emerging body of research on the impact of the pandemic on the CCEE sector has focused on program- and workforce-level responses to the pandemic, such as closures, enrollment, and funding (Barnett et al., 2020; Weiland et al., 2021) and provider well-being (Bassok et al., 2021;

Souto-Manning & Melvin, 2022). A few studies consider how state and local policies issued in response to the COVID-19 pandemic altered CCEE environments, such as instructional practice and interactions between providers and children and providers and families (Pic et al., 2023; Weiland et al., 2021). The perceived impact of the changes experienced by HBCC providers during the pandemic is not fully understood. Changes in cleaning practices, the use of daily monitoring through temperature checks, and virtual instruction have been noted in a few studies that include HBCC providers (Pic et al., 2023; Weiland et al., 2021). Home-based child care providers' experiences, such as daily routines, instructional practices, and material use, have rarely been reported.

To better understand the experiences of HBCC providers, this study was conducted with HBCC providers to understand the following questions:

1. How did HBCC providers perceive the pandemic impacted their daily routines instructional practices?
2. What challenges did HBCC providers experience beyond their day-to-day operations during the early stages of the pandemic?

Frequently, conversations about child care tend to overlook home-based providers, leading to an incomplete grasp of child care issues and experiences. It is notable that home-based child care providers are more likely to be women of color. Hence, within this chapter, we delve into the personal stories of six listed home-based care providers, shedding light on their voices and experiences during the pandemic.

Method

This study draws its sample from a state funded COVID survey of licensed child care providers in the mid-Atlantic region. When the state COVID survey was sent to child care programs during the early months of the pandemic, participants had a choice of indicating their willingness to participate in a follow-up interview to share their personal experiences during the pandemic. Institutional Review Board (IRB) approval was received, and recruitment emails were sent to 53 HBCC providers who indicated their willingness to participate in the survey. Six HBCC providers consented to participate in semi-structured interviews; no compensation was provided for interview participation. A pseudonym was used to protect the participants' confidentiality throughout the chapter. The names mentioned below have been changed for the purposes of this writing and to protect participant identities.

An iterative open-coding approach was used to code and analyze interview transcription data (Corbin & Strauss, 2015; Marshall & Rossman, 2016). Transcript coding was done using Dedoose qualitative coding software (Silver & Lewins, 2014).

During the coding process, three major themes were identified and were developed corresponding subcodes for each theme: changes with physical contact and personal interaction (Hug, no hug, or virtual hug), changes with daily practice (How I survived!), and additional personal and business challenges (Still, it is tough!).

Participants

The participating HBCC providers had considerable experience caring for young children. Participants' years of experience ranged between 14 and 25 years, with a median of 18 years. There were variations in participants' race, age, and years of experience. Three participants in this study identified as Black/African-American and three as White. Study participants ranged in age from 38 years to 62 years of age with a median age of 54.5 years. All participants identified as female and had either completed college credits or a bachelor's degree. Each HBCC provider brought a different background and unique perspective to the shared experience of providing child care during the pandemic.

Bethanne, a married mother whose three children were schooling virtually from home, provided child care for four children between the ages of 2 and 5 years. Her spouse, like many Americans, was also working from home at the time of the COVID-19 pandemic. Bethanne closed temporarily for a few months at the onset of the pandemic and reopened in June; even though one child's parent qualified as an essential worker, they chose to keep their child home. During the 2020-2021 academic year, Bethanne was homeschooling one of her own children during the two-hour nap time window.

Kelly, a single mother, relied on her child care program to pay the bills. She remained open throughout the pandemic, first caring for essential workers' children. The children were 3 and 4 years of age. One enrolled child was full-pay, and the other was a non-paying child of a relative. Ninety-five percent of the children Kelly cared for prior to the onset of the pandemic ceased attending her program. Kelly shifted her hours to better accommodate the two families with children attending her program. Before the pandemic began, her hours were 7:00 AM to 5:00 PM. During the early months of the pandemic, she opened at 7:30 AM and closed at 4:00 PM. At the time of the interview, she was caring for three children.

At the start of the pandemic, Talia closed her child care program when the governor ordered all CCEE programs to be closed unless they were caring for essential workers' children. She reopened in June 2020 and provided care for six children between the ages of 1 and 5 years. Talia's personal health experiences with contracting COVID in the spring of 2020 made her acutely aware of the importance of keeping the children safe once they entered her home. She opted to spend more time indoors with the children rather than risking going outside. Talia felt the risk of someone coming into the yard with COVID-19 was too great to spend time outdoors. Prior to COVID, her program frequently welcomed visitors and members of the community who offered support.

Evangelina did not close during the pandemic. She continued to provide care for three to four children of essential workers during the early months of the pandemic. When additional children were allowed to return, she increased the number of children in her care. At the time of the interview, she was caring for eight children ranging in age between the ages of 2 and 10 years. The children could be heard playing in the background during the interview. Following CDC recommendations, Evangelina required the children in her program to wear masks; during the Zoom interview, she wore a mask.

Prior to the pandemic, Renee cared for nine children ranging in age from 2 to 12 years. At the time of the interview, she was caring for four children ages 7 to 12 years, with children under five years of age enrolled to start in the coming months. Renee remained open throughout the pandemic, first caring for essential workers' children and then adding children back, all of whom were school-age when non-essential workers' children could attend. She mentioned that she shifted her hours four times to accommodate the needs of parents working as essential workers. Children in her care were required to wear masks in accordance with state and CDC guidelines.

Savannah remained open throughout the pandemic, but none of the seven children that were in her care prior to the pandemic were essential workers' children. However, she also did not receive any new children of essential workers during the period when the state mandates only allowed child care programs to operate for essential workers. Once the state allowed child care programs to care for children of non-essential workers, five of the seven children returned. The children that returned ranged in age from 8 months to 11 years.

Interviews with HBCC providers were conducted through Zoom between August and September 2021 and on average lasted approximately 30 minutes. Interviews were recorded with their permission and transcribed verbatim. The Zoom platform allowed for conducting interviews during the time of social distancing. In general, the audio and video quality of the interview was good. At times, interviews had to be momentarily halted to allow the providers to attend to the needs of the children under their care.

Findings

Findings revealed three major themes: 1) "Hug, no hug, or virtual hug" revealing the changes with physical contact and personal interaction, 2) "How I survived!" describing the changes with daily practice, and 3) "Still, it is tough!" unveiling additional personal and business challenges.

Hug, No Hug, or Virtual Hug

The extent of physical contact and close interactions between the HBCC provider and the children in their care, as well as among the children themselves, underwent changes due to the state mandate that required the implementation of social distancing practices. Each provider shared stories about how they altered their interactions with children, having to provide less physical comfort and creating more distance between everyone present. Kelly shared, "I didn't hug the children like I would normally did [sic]...sometimes I would pick them up in spite of their age. I no longer did that." Similarly, Talia mentioned:

> "I've not been able to be as nurturing as I was before. I felt like before I was more hands on. I was more hugging you know, like my arms were open more you know when I'd sit on the floor. Now it's you know, have little spaces and we sit, it's like...I almost feel like sometimes I'm off limits to express that to them...whereas before, when I sat on the floor, especially on their level like if they just wanted a bear hug...I was available for that, but I feel like I had to like pull back because I want to model being able to interact, but at the same time trying to keep my distance."

The inability to provide physical comfort to children who were dealing with their own socio-emotional struggles weighed heavily on Renee. She shared how the school-age children in her care struggled with the deaths of the children's grandparents from COVID and the racial tensions during the summer of 2020:

> "Every single one of the children that I've cared for lost a grandparent…one challenge was helping them deal with that (socio-emotional weight of social distancing) and, unfortunately, the direction that I was given is like do physical activity…doodle and virtual yoga. We did it all, that was not addressing the situation of death…they weren't even finished grieving one death and there comes another…and the racial tension that went on during COVID.

HBCC providers mentioned that adapting to social distancing was a continual struggle despite their best efforts. Kelly expressed, "I tried to social distance as best I could…I do find myself with my mask on hugging them, giving them hugs and high fives." Likewise, Talia shared, "If they just want to run up and hug you know, I take that hug, and I'm like okay, you know let's remember, we have to keep our space." Evangelina shared her struggles with keeping children separated, "The other challenge is like the younger kids keep 'em separate when they're used to playin' together, I had to use a lot of rewards systems as far as explaining to them why they had to be separated."

Providers also discussed issues over mask-wearing, citing confusion caused by changing recommendations and young children's fear of masks. As expressed by Renee, "Now we're back with a mask on so that's going to be a challenge because that's confusing for school-aged children." Bethanne explains how she found mask-wearing challenging for the two-year-old in her care difficult:

> "When they (children) first came back, I was wearing a mask and trying to get them to wear masks, and then the baby came back to me and screamed and cried because she was kind of scared of that and so I said I'm not, I'm not doing this because I'm a home daycare and I'm in my own home and it wasn't going to work for me, so we ditched the masks and everything seemed normal."

Conversely, Evangelina mentioned that the two-year-old in her care was her best mask wearer but she struggled with the older children following the masking requirement, "if his (two-year-old) mask came down, he actually cry wantin' it on so I think the older they got is the harder. I had to keep sayin' please put your mask up, please pull your mask up, please pull your mask up."

Family interactions shifted in response to pandemic restrictions, as parents were no longer allowed to enter the premises. HBCC providers shared that parents and visitors were no longer allowed to enter their homes which altered drop-off and pick-up practices and inhibited daily caregiver-family communication. For example, Savannah shared, "They didn't come in a house during the whole time, well they still don't come in." Similarly, Evangelina stated, "Meet and greet wasn't the same because everybody had to separate…if two parents came together they had to stay out there (the garage), wait until the other ones were (finished with)…their masks…and sanitizer, the temperature check, and then shoes." Evangelina required children to remove their shoes before entering her home to prevent bringing in unwanted germs.

Verbal in-person communication decreased between providers and parents, and emails, text messages; the use of apps also increased. Renee shared that she tried to engage parents in verbal conversation through Zoom to help her understand parents' expectations during this time:

> "They connected, but they didn't participate…I've been involved with these families for years at this point, at least for five or six years…you have your talkers, and you have your non-talkers, but no one was (engaged)…I wanted to know what role they wanted me to play during this COVID."

Although communication with parents shifted for most providers, Kelly expressed that her parents remained informed because she connected to parents through previously established communication channels, "I continued reaching out to the parent and giving them a schedule…still got the schedule every week…got the newsletter, none of that changed."

How I Survived!

Surviving day-to-day while working to ensure children were thriving during the early months of the pandemic required HBCC providers to create new processes and think outside the box. Each HBCC provider shared stories about how they changed the types of instructional materials available to children, adjusted their instructional practices, and recreated their physical space to accommodate COVID-19 mandates and guidelines that required social distancing and increased cleaning. Some HBCC providers also mentioned that they implemented changes in their practices to protect themselves and their children from potential pathogen exposure.

The removal of developmentally appropriate instructional material occurred among all providers. Providers discussed the removal of items such as crayons, dramatic play props such as clothing, utensils, pots, pans, board games, and sensory play materials, including playdough, sand, water, and slime. In Talia's words, "In dramatic play we took the clothing out like the dress up clothing, and we removed… life-like items like the orange juice containers… utensils... because obviously when children are playing, they're actually going to put the utensils in their mouth…pots and pans…and some of the doll babies." Limiting children's access to developmentally appropriate materials created a dilemma for providers. For Evangelina, it also created a storage issue. "I just had to take out stuff because if I didn't take it out, they'd use it and that was a struggle because then I had to make extra storage space." Providers also mentioned reducing activities such as arts and crafts.

Changes in instructional practice occurred within the indoor and outdoor spaces. Kelly discussed how she separated the children but tried to maintain the same activities. She shared, "Basically, they sat apart from one another. We still played almost the same games… it was almost impossible to do social distancing with the two kids as they played." In certain cases, activities that normally took place indoors and involved close proximity were adapted to be conducted outdoors, ensuring that children remained separated from each other. For instance, Evangelina discussed how she transformed indoor board games and circle time activities into the outdoor space: "We would do like ABC runs where they will go find things in the alphabet. They did…virtual tug-of-war, where they had to find things that would make them make a step. If they made a step then the (other) team has a step back…we couldn't use a rope."

Providers also adjusted their curriculum to address the needs of the children. Some of the HBCC providers discussed the increased time they spent on social-emotional learning. Bethanne shared, "There was a lot (more) of the social, emotional piece…kids would actually talk about the virus…there was a lot of things that you could tell were on their mind with what was going on around them, and so we just focused on talking about our feelings." Likewise, Renee expressed her frustration with the lack of support coupled with the increase in the children's social and emotional needs, "I was seein' as far as social, a lot of it was more socially and emotionally. I shared it with my cohorts. I shared it with anybody that was willing to listen... there wasn't any help."

Indoor and outdoor spaces were changed to accommodate the social distancing and cleaning guidelines. Providers shared how they reconfigured furniture and restructured activity areas to provide additional distance between children and between themselves and the children. For instance, Evangelina shared, "I had to get different tables so I could separate them out." Bethanne commented, "I had to bring other little tables into the playroom so we would have more space to do tabletop-type things." During the interview, Savannah provided the researcher with a virtual tour of her spaces, explaining how she subdivided rooms to accommodate school-age children, infants, toddlers, and preschoolers in her care. For example, Savannah narrated,

"That's my dining room. It's my playroom, and this here is my living room where I'm at right now so there's these curtains that are right here that were, that was my barrier, and little kids knew that they couldn't go past there when the curtains are closed…they had to stay over here."

Kelly, whose program remained closed during the time of providing care for essential workers' children, used virtual platforms to maintain connections with families. She recorded herself reading stories one to two times per week and posted them on a group Facebook page; "I just did some stories just to keep in touch with them, but I didn't actually continue with our curriculum, while I was shut down." Three home-based providers who remained open for essential workers' children provided school-aged children Zoom support for school-based instruction. Savannah shared, "When they were doing virtual…I had to rearrange…my house…usually the dining room is for daycare but during that time…I had to set up the dining room as the school for the school agers." Renee also shared her experiences supporting school-age children's virtual learning:

> "All my children were virtual learners from three different schools in two different districts… our days were pretty chaotic… not all the schools went to lunch at the same time… recess became very challenging because I had some children still on Zooms… lunch was scattered within almost a three-hour period."

Home-based child care providers expressed how assisting with virtual teaching for school-age children amplified their workload because of the novel challenge of managing virtual instruction while attending to the needs of younger children in their care or coordinating meals and activities around varying schedules.

Still, it is Tough!

The voice from the HBCC providers revealed that personal health and emotional well-being were influenced by decreases in enrollment, uncertainty about the course of the pandemic, and precarious financial stability. A common sentiment expressed by HBCC in this study was summed up by Kelly's reflection on the challenges posed by the pandemic, "It was challenging mentally and financially... March of 2020 in spite of the fact that me being a Christian, it's almost fear of the unknown...it's the first time I've experienced something of this nature... if I'm not capable of working, then my bills don't get paid...that's when the mental anxiety came in and...you know the human kicks in and the anxiety level is high." Renee expressed how she was exhausted and worn out due to the constant adjustments she had to make to her working hours in order to accommodate the fluctuating schedules of the families she supported. "In the beginning, (my hours) were extended because my essential workers' hours were all changed...they were hospital workers, they were in earlier, so my hours were extended." Renee continued to make adjustments to her working hours as the pandemic continued and the families' needs of care changed:

> "I opened up at 5:30 in the morning two days a week. I closed at 4:00. Two days I closed at 5:00....the month of July and August I closed on Fridays because my parents didn't need me...they were working longer hours....when school started, I changed again. I opened up at 5:30 in the morning and was open till five o'clock two days a week, and three days a week, I was open until 4:00."

Fears experienced during the initial months of the pandemic altered providers' perspectives regarding the age of children they were willing to provide care. Evangelina mentioned, "I would not do infants during COVID. I was too fearful." The availability of physical space with the social distancing requirement also factored into the number of children a provider could enroll. For instance, Bethanne shared, "I actually was supposed to take two more children...because (I) usually do that in the fall...I ended up opting not to take two of the children, just because...the space...that I just didn't have extra rooms."

The increased physical labor (e.g., cleaning, temperature checks, keeping children socially distanced, and extended hours to accommodate parents' needs) emerged as another factor that significantly influenced providers' physical and mental well-being. For instance, Kelly stated, "I just scrub down everything. You know, just took me an hour what normally would take me 30 minutes would take me an hour." Evangelina expressed how the increased cleaning mandate doubled the amount of time she dedicated to cleaning "Any break that I got…I was going to sanitize the table…just washin' all the time…I wanted to just try to hire somebody, but income just wasn't there to hire. So, we had to do what we had to do." Likewise, Renee shared, "I was exhausted, I was opening up at 5:45 in the morning and closing at 5:30 at night and then still had to do all the cleanup. I was going down."

Although the pandemic ushered in uncertainty and financial constraints, HBCC providers were thankful for having their work. For instance, Bethanne shared, "(reopening) actually made even my own social-emotional health better. Getting back into work and having something to do during the day and caring for them and then, you know, interacting with me and with each other." Conversely, she also felt the stress and strain of providing child care in the midst of a global pandemic:

> "I don't even want to even remember some of it…I'm just like 'whoo, close that door' and like let's move on, because it's too painful and hurtful sometimes because it was a lot on, like, just me. I had to be the support person for the parents of the children, for the children, for my own children, and then still have my role as you know, a wife…and so, I think mental health and my own self-care was probably the biggest challenge that I faced."

Lessons Learned

Home-based child care is an important component of the child care system, offering parents a choice in care that more readily meets their needs and preferences. Without HBCC providers, parents would have fewer options for non-traditional hour care, lower child care costs, culturally responsive care, and continuity in care. Providers in this study shared their perspectives on supporting families during the pandemic by providing child care services to families while they navigated the challenges of adhering to state mandates and adjusting their practices in response to the evolving pandemic situation. They shared how they pivoted and shifted to continue to provide safe and quality child care by adapting their daily routines, physical interactions, curriculum, and physical space. Findings of the study are consistent with a review of 63 high-quality studies that noted the impact of the pandemic on child care providers' daily routines, cleaning, and sanitizing practices (Weiland et al., 2021). Similar to other pandemic research that includes HBCC providers, the providers in this study faced challenges with financial stress and personal well-being (Kim et al., 2022; Pic et al., 2023). This study contributes to the existing literature by incorporating the voices of HBCC providers. It highlights their reservations about caring for infants during the pandemic, their interest in seeking external assistance to manage increased cleaning tasks, and their adaptability and flexibility in restructuring their physical environment and adjusting curriculum to address the new demands of providing child care during a pandemic. This study also documents the role HBCC providers played in helping families by adjusting their working hours to meet families changing work hours as the pandemic altered essential workers' hours.

Implications and Policy Recommendations

The HBCC providers in this study continued to provide care with little outside support—financially, physically, or mentally. Home-based child care providers are often an overlooked sector in the child care system, yet they are an integral piece. Their voices need to be heard, especially at a time when listed HBCC providers are on the decline across the U.S. NSECE data comparing 2012 and 2019 collection time points reports a significant decrease in listed family child care (FCC) programs (Datta et al., 2021). This finding is consistent with the National Child Care Licensing Studies that also report the decrease in small FCC homes between 2005 and 2017 (NCECQA, 2020). Ensuring consistent support and funding for HBCC providers, particularly during times of crisis, is a crucial step in stabilizing the HBCC sector and potentially alleviating the ongoing decline.

Obtaining affordable child care, such as the lower cost of home-based child care, is often at the expense of lower wages paid to HBBC providers (U.S. Department of the Treasury, 2021). In general, child care workers are paid lower wages and report experiencing high-stress economic insecurity (Whitebrook et al., 2014), which is more acutely experienced by HBCC providers. The historical lower pay, coupled with pandemic mandates to serve only essential workers and to reduce enrollment, left HBCC providers in this study in precarious financial positions. The unexpected closures, enrollment reductions, and increased costs for cleaning supplies and personal protection equipment due to the pandemic heightened HBCC provider financial instability (Center for the Study of Child Care Employment, 2020). Although federal, state, and local funding was made available for the child care industry, it appears many HBCC providers did not receive funding. None of the HBCC providers in this study mentioned receiving grant monies or funding support. In a study conducted by Bassok and colleagues (2021), of the 74 Virginia family day home teachers surveyed, only 40% received COVID relief funding from federal, state, or local government. Similarly, Kim et al. (2022) noted FCC providers in California suffered income losses due to stay-at-home orders, which decreased enrollment and mandates that allowed care for essential workers' children only. Further, Kim and colleagues (2020) found FCC providers were less likely than their center-based counterparts to receive stimulus funding. The voices of the HBCC providers in this study support prior research that documents discrepancies in the child care sector based on program type and funding (Whitebrook et al., 2018). It is imperative that HBCCs be fully included in funding and financial support when natural disasters and global events such as the pandemic occur. The voices of the HBCC providers underscore the importance of stable funding, especially in a time of global crisis, and highlight the need to ensure funding reaches HBCC providers.

Additional support for HBCC providers should include access to providing children and families with comprehensive services and supports—informal and formal services that support the whole-child and whole-family outcomes (Melvin et al., 2023). The HBCC providers in this study were providing families with support by providing masks, advice and guidance, and flexible schedules. However, these providers were not receiving the support they desired to help them address the social and emotional needs of the children in their care and the financial assistance to help with the increased cleaning and the loss of income due to decreased enrollment and program closure. Melvin and colleagues (2023) suggest the use of HBCC networks and government agencies to provide comprehensive services and supports, such as the ones employed in Head Start programs, as a promising initiative that can bolster the HBCC sector. Access to comprehensive services and support could have provided the HBCC providers in this study with access to mental health consultants, social workers, financial assistance, and strategies for responding to families in crisis.

This study examined HBCC providers' perspectives and experiences on the impact of the pandemic on their practices during the early months of COVID. HBCC providers encountered many challenges, yet they were able to adapt their daily practices to meet the needs of the children even with little support from the state and federal government. It is important to consider HBCC providers' voices and their unique needs when policy decisions are made during times of crisis, such as the pandemic.

References

Ali, U., Herbst, C. M., & Makridis, C. A. (2021). The impact of COVID-19 on the U.S. child care market: Evidence from stay-at-home orders. *Economics of Education Review, 82*. https://doi.org/10.1016/j.econedurev.2021.102094

Banghart, P. (2022). *Factors that influence families' search for child care and early education.* OPRE Report #2022-70. Office of Planning, Research, and Evaluation, Administration for Children and Families, U.S. Department of Health and Human Services. https://eric.ed.gov/?id=ED621233

Barnett, S., Jung, K., & Nores, M. (2020). *Young children's home learning and preschool participation experiences during the pandemic: NIEER 2020 preschool learning activities survey.* (Technical report and selected findings). National Institute for Early Education Research. https://nieer.org/research-report/young-childrens-home-learning-and-preschool-participation-experiences-during-the-pandemic

Bassok, D., Weisner, K., Doromal, J. B., & Michie, M. (2021). *Virginia's family day homes in the early months of COVID-19: Lessons from two waves of the PDG B-5 workforce survey.* https://files.elfsightcdn.com/022b8cb9-839c-4bc2-992e-cefccb8e877e/5ebe3729-c47d-4559-92f8-80a0a38016f4.pdf

Center for the Study of Child Care Employment. (2020). *California child care in crisis: COVID-19 impacts escalate as California reopens.* Data Snapshot. University of California, Berkeley. https://cscce.berkeley.edu/publications/data-snapshot/california-child-care-in-crisis-covid-19/

Chaudry, A., Henly, J., & Meyers, M. (2010). *ACF-OPRE White Paper. Conceptual Frameworks for Child Care Decision-Making*. Office of Planning, Research and Evaluation, Administration for Children and Families, U.S. Department of Health and Human Services. https://eric.ed.gov/?id=ED517547

Corbin, J. M., & Strauss, A. L. (2015). *Basics of qualitative research: Techniques and procedures for developing grounded theory* (4th ed.). SAGE.

Crawford, A., Vaughn, K. A., Guttentag, C. L., Varghese, C., Oh, Y., & Zucker, T. A. (2021). "Doing what I can, but I got no magic wand:" A snapshot of early childhood educator experiences and efforts to ensure quality during the COVID-19 pandemic. *Early Childhood Education Journal, 49*(5), 829-840. https://doi.org/10.1007/s10643-021-01215-z

Cui, J., & Natzke, L. (2021). *Early childhood program participation: 2019* (NCES 2020-075REV), National Center for Education Statistics, Institute of Education Sciences, U.S. Department of Education. Washington, DC. http://nces.ed.gov/pubsearch/pubsinfo.asp?pubid=2020075REV

Datta, A. R., Milesi, C., Srivastava, S., & Zapata-Gietl, C. (2021). *Home-based early care and education providers in 2012 and 2019: Counts and characteristics*. Chartbook. National Survey of Early Care & Education. OPRE Report 2021-85. Administration for Children & Families. https://www.acf.hhs.gov/opre/report/home-based-early-care-and-education-providers-2012-and-2019-counts-and-characteristics

Delaware Department of Service for Children, Youth & Their Families. (2020, March). *Additional requirements for DSCYF-designated emergency child care sites.* https://governor.delaware.gov/wpcontent/uploads/sites/24/2020/03/DSCYF-Emergency-Child-Care-Site-Requirements.pdf

Ferreira van Leer, K., & Coley, R. L. (2023). Early childhood education decision-making among Latinx foreign-born parents in the United States: A culturally-informed model of decision-making. *Children and Youth Services Review, 151*, 107046–. https://doi.org/10.1016/j.childyouth.2023.107046

Forry, N. D., Tout, K., Rothenberg, L., Sandstrom, H., & Vesely, C. (2013). *Child Care Decision-Making Literature Review*. OPRE Brief 2013-45. Office of Planning, Research and Evaluation, Administration for Children and Families, U.S. Department of Health and Human Services. https://www.acf.hhs.gov/opre/report/child-care-decision-making-literature-review

Hill, Z., Ekyalongo, Y., Paschall, K., Madill, R., & Halle, T. (2021). *A demographic comparison of the listed home-based workforce and the children in their care.* OPRE Report #2020-128, Office of Planning, Research, and Evaluation, Administration for Children and Families, U.S. Department of Health and Human Services. https://www.acf.hhs.gov/sites/default/files/documents/opre/demographic%20comparison%20liste.pdf

Kim, Y., Montoya, E., Doocy, S., Austin, L. J. E., & Whitebook, M. (2022). Impacts of COVID-19 on the early care and education sector in California: Variations across program types. *Early Childhood Research Quarterly, 60*, 348–362. https://doi.org/10.1016/j.ecresq.2022.03.004

Marshall, C., & Rossman, G. B. (2016). *Designing Qualitative Research* (6th ed.). SAGE.

Melvin, S.A., Reinoso, L., Bromer, J. & Porter, T. (2023). *Unpacking comprehensive services and supports in family child care: The role of networks.* Erikson Institute. https://www.erikson.edu/wp-content/uploads/2023/07/EI_NetworkStudyCSS_Brief_JULY2023.pdf

National Center on Early Childhood Quality Assurance (NCECQA). (2020). *Addressing the decreasing number of family child care providers in the United States.* Administration for Children and Families, Office of Child Care, U.S. Department of Health and Human Services. https://child careta.acf.hhs.gov/resource/addressing-decreasing-number-family-child-care-providers-united-states

National Survey of Early Care and Education Project Team. (2014). *Household search for and perceptions of early care and education: Initial findings from the National Survey of Early Care and Education (NSECE)* (OPRE Report No. 2014-55a). Washington, DC: Office of Planning, Research and Evaluation, Administration for Children and Families, U.S. Department of Health and Human Services. https://www.acf.hhs.gov/sites/default/files/documents/opre/brief_hh_search_and_perceptions_to_opre_10022014.pdf

National Survey of Early Care and Education Project Team (2015). *Fact Sheet: Provision of Early Care and Education during Non-Standard Hours.* (OPRE Report No. 2015-44). Washington, DC: Office of Planning, Research and Evaluation, Administration for Children and Families, U.S. Department of Health and Human Services. Available at http://www.acf.hhs.gov/programs/opre/research/project/national-survey-of-early-care-andeducation-nsece-2010-2014

National Survey of Early Care and Education Project Team (2016). *Characteristics of Home-based Early Care and Education Providers: Initial Findings from the National Survey of Early Care and Education.* OPRE Report #2016-13, Office of Planning, Research and Evaluation, Administration for Children and Families, U.S. Department of Health and Human Services. https://www.acf.hhs.gov/opre/report/characteristics-home-based-early-care-and-education-providers-initial-findings-national

New Jersey Department of Children and Families. (2020). *Guidance for New Jersey child care facilities on COVID-19 related health and safety requirements.*

Children and families' Office of child care Licensing. https://www.nj.gov/dcf/news/Final.CC.Health.and.Safety.Standards.pdf

Paschall, K. (2019). *Nearly 30 percent of infants and toddlers attend home-based child care as their primary arrangement*. Child Trends. https://www.childtrends.org/blog/nearly-30-percent-of-infants-and-toddlers-attend-home-based-child-care-as-their-primary-arrangement

Pattnaik, J., & Lopez, M. (2023). Financial challenges of family child care providers during the COVID-19 Pandemic: A phenomenological study. *Early Childhood Education Journal*, 1-15. https://doi.org/10.1007/s10643-023-01477-9

Pic, A., Han, M., Whitaker, A., & Barnes, T. N. (2023). Early childhood educators' perspectives on the impact of COVID-19 on child care. *Social Education Research*, 194–208. https://doi.org/10.37256/ser.4220232529

Schilder, D. K., Willenborg, Lou, C., Knowles, S., & Jaramillo, J. (2021). *Comparing potential demand for nontraditional-hour child care and planned policies across states.* Urban Institute. https://www.urban.org/sites/default/files/publication/104601/comparing-potential-demand-for-nontraditional-hour-child-care-and-planned-policies-across-states.pdf

Silver, C., & Lewins, A. (2014). *Using software in qualitative research: A step-by-step guide* (2nd ed.). SAGE.

Souto-Manning, M., & Melvin, S. A. (2022). Early childhood teachers of color in New York City: Heightened stress, lower quality of life, declining health, and compromised sleep amidst COVID-19. *Early Childhood Research Quarterly, 60*, 34–48. https://doi.org/10.1016/j.ecresq.2021.11.005

Theilheimer, R. (2006). Molding to the children: Primary caregiving and continuity of care. *Zero to Three, 26*(3), 50-54.

United States Department of Treasury. (2021). *Economics of child care supply in the United States.* White Paper. https://home.treasury.gov/system/files/136/The-Economics-of-child care-Supply-09-14-final.pdf

Weber, R. (2011). *Understanding parents' child care decision-making: A foundation for policy making*. OPRE 2011-12. Office of Planning, Research and Evaluation, Administration for Children and Families, U.S. Department of Health and Human Services.

https://www.acf.hhs.gov/opre/report/understanding-parents-child-care-decision-making-foundation-child-care-policy-making

Weiland, C., Greenberg, E., Bassok, D., Markowitz, A., Guerrero Rosada, P., Luetmer, G., Gomez, C., Johnson, A., Jones-Harden, B., Maier, M., McCormick, M., Morris, P., Nores, M., Phillips, D., & Snow, C. (2021). *Historic crisis, historic opportunity: Using evidence to mitigate the effects of the COVID-19 crisis on young children and early care and education programs.* (Policy Brief). University of Michigan Education Policy Initiative and Urban Institute. https://edpolicy.umich.edu/files/EPI-UICOVID%20Synthesis%20Brief%20June%202021.pdf

About the Contributing Authors:

Annette Pic, Ph.D., is a researcher at the Delaware Institute for Excellence in Early Childhood (DIEEC), University of Delaware. She is a methodology lead for the National Early Care and Education Workforce Center, Research and Knowledge Development team. She also works on state-level funded projects centered on improving early care and education quality and access. Her research interests include early childhood policy and systems and equitable access to early care and education for families experiencing homelessness with young children.

Myae Han, Ph.D. is a Professor in the Department of Human Development and Family Sciences at the University of Delaware, a past president of The Association for the Study of Play (TASP) and Early Education and Child Development Special Interest Group (SIG) at the American Educational Research Association. Her research includes play-based intervention, early language and literacy development, and professional development of early childhood teachers.

Section III

The Post-COVID Era, the "New Normal," and Recommendations for the Future of Early Childhood Education

Chapter 8
Changes in the Perception, Evaluation, and Appreciation of the Early Childhood Education Profession

The COVID-19 pandemic has had far-reaching effects on various aspects of society, including the field of early childhood education (ECE). As the world grappled with the challenges brought about by the virus, the perception and evaluation of the ECE profession underwent significant transformations. This chapter explores the changes related to how the ECE profession was perceived and evaluated during the COVID-19 health crisis.

In several countries around the world, ECE programs are part of the official education system, ECE professionals are valued and compensated the same way school teachers are, and they also enjoy the same benefits. The ECE programs are universal and publicly funded. This is the case in Belgium, Denmark, France, Hungary, Iceland, Israel, Norway, Spain and the United Kingdom where preschool children have the highest level of enrollment (Organization for Economic Cooperation and Development, 2019). In contrast, the United States (U.S.) has a largely underfunded and fractured ECE system with a wide range of programs and services designed to support the development of young children. The system is characterized by a combination of public and private providers, various funding sources, and a lack of a unified national framework (Kagan & Kauerz, 2015). Some key components of the early childhood system in the U.S. include state pre-kindergarten programs, child care and home-based programs, private preschools, and public kindergartens and public schools.

This diversity in programming also results in diversity in compensation and appreciation for ECE professionals. For example, there are many in society who have often viewed ECE programs as daycares and not as educational institutions of learning. As such, the educators in those classrooms are also seen as not needing the same recognition and compensation as Kindergarten - Grade 12 educators (McLean et al., 2021). Yet, private and public preschool programs typically have a strong educational focus, aiming to prepare children for kindergarten and beyond. They often follow a structured curriculum that focuses on early academic skills, socialization, and school readiness. The educators in these classrooms have the academic background of a K-12 teacher, yet their salary varies drastically (McLean et al., 2021).

On the other hand, child care centers are viewed as institutions that provide comprehensive care and supervision for children while their parents or guardians are at work or otherwise occupied. There is typically more flexibility regarding the educational level needed for this position. Yet, their positions are critical to society and not compensated as such.

Although there is a difference between the several types of programs that existed during the COVID pandemic, many of these roles became blurred as all ECE educators needed to take on non-teaching tasks, including emotional support, family collaboration, COVID hygiene protocol, and technological support.

Appreciation of the Complexity of ECE: Teacher and Parent Perceptions

A survey interviewing teachers and parents highlighted the attitudes participants developed towards early childhood education, the role of educators, and the need for highly trained professionals to teach young children. Historically, the early childhood field has received less respect than other fields, even within education. The common belief is that for most part early childhood is just child care and that people without specialized training can do it effectively.

During the pandemic, however, parents struggled to keep their children occupied and engaged in activities. Furthermore, parents faced obstacles when trying to educate their children or to make sure their learning did not suffer. The pandemic offered a unique window to study attitudes towards teaching young children. When children spent most of their time at home and adults struggled to keep children entertained and educated, many asked themselves what activities were developmentally appropriate? How much time does an educator spend preparing curriculum? How do we keep young children engaged?

Parent and Teacher Survey

During the spring of 2020, a group of parents and early childhood educators participated in a short survey. The survey included parents and educators enrolled in a variety of early childhood settings, such as private and public preschools and child care programs (for more information on data collection and participants, please see Chapter 2). The survey asked them to rate each statement below with "Strongly Disagree," "Disagree," "Agree," and "Strongly Agree."

1. Teaching young children is easy and anyone can do it.
2. Teaching young children takes a substantial amount of planning time.
3. Teaching young children involves understanding young children's interests and needs.
4. Teaching young children involves understanding developmentally appropriate practices (DAP).
5. Teaching young children involves understanding appropriate curriculum and resources.
6. Teaching young children involves understanding how to assess learning and development.
7. Teaching young children involves understanding how to engage young children in learning.
8. Teaching young children involves understanding how to manage behavior with positive interactions.

9. I believe that ECE is adequately valued in our society.
10. I believe people appreciate ECE teachers more now that children are mostly home.

The responses to the statements were rated as followed: Strongly Disagree = 1, Disagree = 2, Agree = 3, and Strongly Agree = 4. Table 1 summarizes the average rating for each of the statements.

Means	*M* Teachers	*M* Families	*M* Total
Anyone can teach ECE	1.62	1.82	1.77
Take time/planning	3.22	3.45	3.59
Understanding interests and needs	3.88	3.64	3.77
Understanding DAP	3.90	3.82	3.86
Understanding curriculum and resources	3.85	1.92	2.91
Understanding DAP in Assessment	3.90	1.92	2.94
Engage children	3.92	3.45	3.69
Manage behaviors with positive interactions	3.92	3.64	3.79
ECE adequately valued	2.53	3.77	3.13
More appreciative since COVID-19	3.44	1.86	2.67

Table 8.1 *Average Rating for Each Statement*

(Strongly Disagree = 1, Disagree = 2, Agree = 3 and Strongly Agree = 4)

Survey Responses

The results shown in Table 1 highlight that most participants disagree with the statement "Teaching young children is easy and anyone can do it." At the same time, the majority of participants agreed that the profession involves a high level of complexity when it comes time for planning, understanding young children's needs and interests, understanding how to engage young children in learning, and managing behaviors in positive ways. This points at support and appreciation of the ECE profession during the pandemic. Nevertheless, educators and parents differed in their perception of the complexity of the profession in several ways. These differences are presented in Table 8.2.

		Sum of Squares	*df*	Mean Square	F	*p*
Anyone can teach ECE students	Between Groups	.99	1	.99	1.21	.274
	Within Groups	84	103	.82		
	Total	85	104			
Time and planning	Between Groups	1.9	1	1.9	5.94	.017
	Within Groups	33	103	.33		
	Total	35	104			
Interests and Needs	Between Groups	1.5	1	1.5	8.32	.005
	Within Groups	19	103	.18		
	Total	21	104			
Understanding DAP	Between Groups	.19	1	.19	1.36	.246
	Within Groups	14	103	.13		
	Total	14	104			
Curriculum and Resources	Between Groups	98	1	98	1.61	.000
	Within Groups	63	103	.61		
	Total	160	104			

		Sum of Squares	*df*	Mean Square	F	*p*
DAP in Assessment	Between Groups	103	1	103	1.83	.000
	Within Groups	58	103	.57		
	Total	162	104			
Engage Children	Between Groups	5.9	1	6.0	25	.000
	Within Groups	24	103	.24		
	Total	30	104			
Manage Behavior	Between Groups	2.0	1	2.0	12	.001
	Within Groups	17	103	.17		
	Total	19	104			
Profession is Valued	Between Groups	40	1	40	47	.000
	Within Groups	87	103	.84		
	Total	126	104			
Appreciated More	Between Groups	66	1	66	92	.000
	Within Groups	73	103	.71		
	Total	139	104			

Table 8.2 *ANOVA Results for Comparing Responses of Teachers and Families*

ANOVA tests were performed to determine if there were statistically significant differences in average perceived views of ECE and teaching in several respondents (teachers vs. family). According the results presented in Table 2, "Anyone can teach ECE students" was not significant [$F(1, 103) = 1.21$, $p = .274$]; "Understanding DAP" was also not significant [$F(1, 103) = 1.36$, $p = .246$], suggesting that families and teachers viewed these two aspects of the profession very similarly.

However, the results on ANOVA show significant differences among teachers and parents, pointing at the gap of appreciation for the complexity of the profession. Teachers' average rating for the following items were higher than for families, indicating that teachers thought the field is more complex and demanding than parents did. For example, teachers were significantly more likely than parents to agree with "Teaching young children takes a substantial amount of planning time" [$F(1, 103) = 5.94$, $p = .017$]. Similarly, teachers were significantly more likely than parents to agree with "Teaching young children involves understanding young children's interest and needs" as $F(1, 103) = 8.32$, $p = .005$. Furthermore, teachers expressed significantly higher levels of agreements with the statement "Teaching young children involves understanding appropriate curriculum and resources" [$F(1, 103) = 1.61$, $p = .000$] and "teaching young children involves understanding how to assess learning and development" [$F(1, 103) = 1.83$, $p = .000$]. Teachers also rated the need for ECE teachers to be able to engage young children higher [$F(1, 103) = .25$, $p = .000$]; they also rated the ability to manage children's behavior higher than parents[$F(1, 103) = .12$, $p = .001$]. Lastly, parents were significantly more likely to think that the ECE is adequately valued in our society [$F(1, 103) = .47$, $p = .000$]. Teachers were significantly more likely to agree that the value for ECE has increased during the COVID-19 pandemic [$F(1, 103) = .92$, $p = .000$].

Interpretation of Survey Findings

The data gathered through the survey conveys important information. The ECE profession is complex and requires a skillful and trained professional with knowledge and understanding of all domains in child development and developmentally appropriate practices (DAP).

Teachers support cognitive development through understanding of DAP curriculum and resources, and teachers assess learning and development through the use of DAP assessment tools. Furthermore, the ECE professional is responsible for promoting motivation for learning by understanding children's needs, interests, and engagement. In addition, teachers need to be skillful in fostering social development through guidance and positive interactions.

Yet, there is a gap in appreciation of the demands of the job, and ECE parents are less likely to recognize the complexity of proficiencies required to fill the role of an early childhood educator than teachers. Most teachers have scored the items related to planning curriculum, understanding DAP, assessment and curriculum resources, engaging young children and managing behaviors higher than parents did, indicating that parents don't always appreciate the extent of work that goes into educating young children.

Despite this gap, parents were more likely to think that the role of ECE educators is appropriately appreciated in our society, while teachers were less likely to think this is the case. Similarly, teachers were more likely to think that the appreciation for the role of ECE educators had increased during the pandemic.

Changes in Early Childhood Professionals' Status

Nevertheless, the pandemic brought about several changes in the perception and status of the ECE professional. Some of these changes contributed positively, while other changes added new demands on an already stressed task force. The role of the ECE professional expanded, but the appreciation and compensation has not always matched the new definitions of the role. The COVID-19 pandemic brought about significant changes in the perception and evaluation of the early childhood education profession. Early childhood educators were recognized as essential workers, and their contributions to child development and family support were valued more than ever before

(Quinn et al., 2022). The evaluation criteria expanded to include adaptability to remote learning, implementation of health and safety measures, provision of emotional support, and dedication to professional growth.

Recognition of Essential Status

One of the changes the pandemic brought about was the recognition of early childhood professionals as essential workers. The pandemic shed light on the essential role played by early childhood educators in supporting children's development and enabling parents to continue working (Quinn et al., 2022). As schools temporarily closed, the importance of ECE professionals in providing care, education, and emotional support became evident. The perception of the ECE profession shifted, with educators being recognized as essential workers deserving of respect and fair compensation. While many early childhood programs closed at some point due to the pandemic several ECE workers, especially those in child care centers, were considered essential workers (Weiland et al., 2021).

The recognition as essential workers became a double-sided sword, as it resulted in new responsibilities and, at the same time, new risks. Similarly to other service fields, many of the ECE workers in the U.S. were predominantly women of color (Weiland et al., 2021). While public school teachers taught remotely, ECE teachers went back to work. During this time, educators experienced significant changes, such as an increase in the number of students and ages they were responsible for supervising and changes in the number of hours and pay (Weiland et al., 2021). Historically, ECE educators were low-paid and could not always afford to have good healthcare coverage (McLean et al., 2021), yet were required to report to work while vaccines or treatment for COVID-19 were not readily available. With increased health risks, the responsibilities of ECE professionals expanded in unprecedented ways.

New Responsibilities and New Risks: Healthcare

During the pandemic, ECE teachers became tasked with ensuring the health and safety of young children. Early childhood educators were tasked with implementing rigorous hygiene protocols, promoting social distancing among children, and managing anxieties related to the virus. Their ability to create a safe and supportive environment became a crucial aspect of their evaluation. While ECE educators were tasked with this protocol, they faced poor healthcare benefits to support them during the pandemic. In fact, ECE educators are not only underpaid in the U.S., but also have poor healthcare benefits (McLean et al., 2021).

Many early childhood education programs, particularly those in publicly funded settings or nonprofit organizations, operate on limited budgets. As a result, they may face financial constraints when it comes to providing robust healthcare benefits. Lower wages made it more challenging for educators to afford comprehensive healthcare coverage or contribute towards higher premiums. In some cases, ECE educators may not have strong union representation or collective bargaining power to negotiate for better benefits. Healthcare benefits can also vary depending on the state, the specific educational setting (public, private, or nonprofit), and the employer. Differences in state regulations, funding, and priorities can contribute to disparities in healthcare benefits for ECE educators.

New Responsibilities and New Risks: Emotional Wellbeing and Mental Health

The COVID-19 crisis brought increased stress and anxiety to children and families. Early childhood educators played a vital role in providing emotional support, stability, and a sense of normalcy during these challenging times (Watts & Pattnaik, 2023). They had to develop new strategies to address children's fears and anxieties, promote mental well-being, and collaborate with families to navigate the emotional impact of the pandemic. The evaluation of ECE professionals encompassed their ability to support children's socio-emotional development and maintain strong partnerships with families.

Consequently, ECE educators struggled as many settings lacked a support system to guide educators' well-being during the pandemic. Educators experienced increased stress and anxiety. The pandemic introduced uncertainty, fear, and increased workloads for ECE educators. The need to adapt to new teaching methods, implement health and safety protocols, and manage the well-being of young children in a changing environment added to their stress levels. This heightened anxiety and stress that had negatively affected their emotional well-being (Watts & Pattnaik, 2023). Their concerns for themselves and their families' health and safety also played a critical role in the well-being of ECE educators. ECE educators were on the front lines, providing care and education to young children who may not have fully understood or followed safety guidelines. This heightened their concerns about contracting and transmitting the virus; fear of exposure to the virus, and its potential impact on their health and the health of their families, contributed to increased stress levels.

Increased work demands and burnout during the pandemic were at their highest point. The pandemic led to increased work demands as ECE educators had to adapt their teaching methods to remote or hybrid learning, implement new health and safety protocols, and navigate the challenges of supporting young children's social and emotional well-being during a time of crisis (Farewell et al., 2023). The added workload and pressure led to burnout and exhaustion, impacting ECE educators' emotional well-being (Farewell et al., 2023). Financial, food, and healthcare insecurities affected 60% of ECE educators, adding to their emotional stress levels (McLean et al., 2021; McCormack et al., 2020).

ECE educators lacked access to sufficient resources, training, and guidance to effectively navigate the challenges posed by the pandemic. This lack of support and guidance exacerbated the feelings of frustration, helplessness, and emotional strain. Educators reported spending additional time on non-teaching tasks, having time pressures that compromised their educational philosophies, and feeling overworked due to the increased turnover in the field (McLean et al., 2021).

New Responsibilities and New Demands: Professional Development and Resilience

The pandemic highlighted the importance of ongoing professional development and adaptability in the ECE profession (Callaway-Cole et al., 2021). Educators needed to upskill themselves in areas such as technology integration, trauma-informed practices, and online pedagogy. The evaluation of ECE professionals encompassed their ability to continuously learn, adapt to changing circumstances, and demonstrate resilience in the face of adversity.

With the closure of physical classrooms, early childhood educators faced the unprecedented challenge of transitioning to remote learning environments. This sudden shift required them to quickly acquire digital skills, create engaging online content, and maintain meaningful connections with young children and their families (Callaway-Cole et al., 2021). The evaluation of ECE professionals expanded to include their ability to adapt to virtual platforms and facilitate remote learning effectively. Teacher education programs adopted these changes while trying to keep high professional standards for students in fieldwork and practicum courses (Callaway-Cole et al., 2021).

While collaboration with families in the early childhood field has been an integral part of teaching and learning, the pandemic underscored the importance of strong partnerships between ECE educators and families. Educators had to maintain regular communication with parents/guardians, provide resources and guidance for supporting children's learning at home, and ensure a collaborative approach to navigate the challenges of remote or hybrid learning.

What Changed

There are several aspects in the early childhood field that changed post-COVID. Nonetheless, there are many systemic changes that remain in the workforce. Educators and students transitioned to in-person learning as the conditions improved around them. Each setting reopened to full or partial in-person learning. Educators began to slowly and intentionally re-introduce children to direct social interactions and facilitate hands-on learning experiences. The return to in-person learning meant educators needed to navigate a "new normal" - for example, the need to maintain ongoing health and safety measures. ECE educators continued to implement health and safety measures to ensure the well-being of children, staff, and families. This included adhering to hygiene protocols, monitoring symptoms, and following any specific guidelines or recommendations from health authorities.

One important change in practice was the introduction of digital media. Although teaching and learning returned to the traditional in-person mode, there has been a major incorporation of technology in all grades, including in preschool (Hu et al., 2021). The use of technology that emerged during the pandemic, such as the use of online learning platforms and digital resources, was integrated into ECE classrooms (Hu et al., 2021). Educators leveraged technology to enhance teaching practices, support individualized learning, and promote family engagement through digital communication tools (Hu et al., 2021).

Another change has been the focus on emotional well-being. The pandemic highlighted the importance of addressing children's mental health. ECE educators placed increased emphasis on creating supportive and nurturing environments, implementing social-emotional learning strategies, and promoting resilience and mental health among young children (Silver & Zinsser, 2022). ECE educators recognized the need for ongoing professional development to adapt to evolving educational practices and meet the unique needs of children. Opportunities for training and learning focused on trauma-informed care, equity and inclusion, emerging teaching methodologies, and strategies to support children who may have experienced disruption due to the pandemic (Silver & Zinsser, 2022).

The pandemic further underscored the critical role of ECE educators and the need for increased support, resources, and recognition. Nonetheless, there needs to be further advocacy efforts to secure funding, improve compensation and benefits, and advocate for policies that prioritize the well-being of ECE educators and the quality of early childhood education - in addition to increasing emphasis on ensuring equitable access to early childhood education for all, addressing learning gaps, and providing support to vulnerable populations.

ECE educators have continued to foster collaborations and partnerships with families, community organizations, and other stakeholders to enhance children's learning experiences.

Engaging families and communities in the educational process can support children's holistic development and create a more comprehensive support system. The pandemic necessitated a higher degree of flexibility and adaptability among ECE educators. Post-COVID, these skills remain valuable as educators continue to navigate uncertainties, changing circumstances, and emerging educational needs.

What Remains

Despite the many challenges faced by the ECE field and the systemic need for change, governments, policymakers, and educational institutions have not prioritized increased investment in ECE programs. Adequate funding can support improved infrastructure, resources, professional development opportunities for educators, and equitable access to high-quality early childhood education for all children. There has been no change after the COVID-19 pandemic.

Despite the fact that ECE educators were recognized as essential workers, enhanced compensation and benefits for educators remained the same after the pandemic. It appears that early childhood educators' crucial role in society was recognized but not compensated. There haven't been changes by policymakers to improve their compensation and benefits in the U.S. (McLean et al., 2021), and discussions regarding fair and competitive wages, comprehensive healthcare benefits, and retirement plans by policymakers have not been taken seriously. Making these changes can attract and retain skilled educators, promoting stability and quality within the field.

Similarly, the ECE system remains as fragmented as ever with inconsistencies regarding quality standards, teacher accreditation, curriculum guidelines, professional compensation, and funding across the several programs that comprise the field. In the post-COVID era, it is imperative to develop policies that ensure equitable access to early childhood education provided by well-compensated professionals.

Conclusion

The pandemic allowed ECE educators to be viewed as an integral part of society as child care is key for working families across the U.S. Survey data points at a gap in appreciation for the profession as whole and the need to educate the public into understanding the complex roles of ECE professionals. Additional literature highlights new demands brought upon early childhood educators during the pandemic. As the responsibilities and risks changed, the compensation and recognition remained the same.

In order to change many of the shortcomings highlighted during the pandemic, it is imperative that action is taken during this post-COVID time, as the issues are still relevant, and as there is newfound societal support and for ECE educators. As society moves forward, the lessons learned during the pandemic can help shape a stronger and more resilient ECE profession capable of addressing future challenges, providing high-quality care, and offering a more dynamic education to young children. The next chapter will discuss several changes needed in the profession that were highlighted by COVID-19.

References

Callaway-Cole, L., Kimble, A. Maintaining Professional Standards in Early Childhood Teacher Preparation: Evaluating Adaptations to Fieldwork-Based Experiences During COVID-19. *Early Childhood Educ J, 49*, 841–853 (2021). https://doi.org/10.1007/s10643-021-01227-9

Farewell, C. V., Quinlan, J., Gonzales, L., & Puma, J. (2023). Changes in demands and resources faced by the early childhood education workforce due to COVID-19. *Journal of Early Childhood Research, 21*(1), 63-75. https://doi.org/10.1177/1476718X221136463

Hu, X., Chiu, M. M., Leung, W. M. V., & Yelland, N. (2021). Technology integration for young children during COVID-19: Towards future online teaching. *British journal of educational technology : journal of the Council for Educational Technology, 52*(4), 1513–1537. https://doi.org/10.1111/bjet.13106

Kagan, L., & Kauerz, K. (2015). *Early childhood systems: Transforming early learning*. Teachers College Press.

McCormack G., Avery C., Spitzer A.K.L., Chandra A. (2020). Economic vulnerability of households with essential workers. *JAMA.* 2020;324:388–390. doi: 10.1001/jama.2020.11366.

McLean, C., Austin, L.J.E., Whitebook, M., & Olson, K.L. (2021). Early Childhood Workforce Index – 2020. Berkeley, CA: Center for the Study of Child Care Employment, University of California, Berkeley. Retrieved from https://cscce.berkeley.edu/workforce-index-2020/report-pdf/

OECD (2019), *Education at a Glance 2019: OECD Indicators*, OECD Publishing, Paris, https://doi.org/10.1787/f8d7880d-en

Quinn E.L., Stover, B, Otten J.J., Seixas, N. (2022) Early Care and Education Workers' Experience and Stress during the COVID-19 Pandemic. *International Journal of Environmental Research and Public Health 19*(5):2670. https://doi.org/10.3390/ijerph19052670

Silver, H. C., & Zinsser, K. M. (2022). Lessons for the future: Supporting the social-emotional needs of children, families, and educators in Head Start during the COVID-19 pandemic. *Translational Issues in Psychological Science, 8*(3), 362–374. https://doi.org/10.1037/tps0000335

Watts, R., Pattnaik, J. Perspectives of Parents and Teachers on the Impact of the COVID-19 Pandemic on Children's Socio-Emotional Well-Being. *Early Childhood Educ J, 51,* 1541–1552 (2023). https://doi.org/10.1007/s10643-022-01405-3

Weiland C., Greenberg E., Bassok D., Markowitz A., Rosada P.G., Luetmer G., Abenavoli R., Gomez C., Johnson A., Jones-Harden B., et al. (2021). *Historic Crisis, Historic Opportunity: Using Evidence to Mitigate the Effects of the COVID-19 Crisis on Young Children and Early Care and Education Programs.* Gerald R Ford School of Public Policy, University of Michigan and Urban Institute; Ann Arbor, MI, USA.

Chapter 9
Lessons Learned and Recommendations for Early Childhood Education Policy

The early years play a critical role in a child's learning and development. Children begin learning at birth and proceed to develop at a rapid pace through their early years. Their respective environments, supports, and relationships all have a profound effect. Development in early childhood is not only rapid but also cumulative; early learning provides a foundation on which later learning is constructed. High quality learning environments support continued development achievements. The adults who guide that learning and provide care and education for young children bear a great responsibility to their health, growth, development, learning, and building of social and emotional foundations for life-long learning (Institute of Medicine and National Research Council, 2015). This responsibility has been highlighted during the COVID-19 health crisis.

Early childhood educators in the U.S. work in a variety of settings with diverse circumstances, such as homes, child care centers, private and publicly funded preschools, family-based centers, and district schools (Institute of Medicine and National Research Council, 2015). A growing public understanding for the importance of early childhood education is needed to change attitudes toward the profession and spark policy and investments. Currently, the sophistication and complexity of the professional roles required for working with young children are not recognized; this is reflected in policies, compensation, and working conditions. Those who work with young children are not always acknowledged as a unified workforce identified by their knowledge, skills, and preparation (Institute of Medicine and National Research Council, 2015).

The following recommendations are based on the lessons learned during COVID-19. The challenges encountered during the COVID-19 health crises are not new. For too long, policies for the early childhood education (ECE) field have been making do with existing systems instead of focusing on what is needed and committing to strategies necessary to achieve them. Substantive changes need to be implemented to elevate the perception of ECE professionals and the status of the workforce.

Changes should be driven by the science of early learning and child development as well as supported by policymakers and a society that understands the complex and important role of the ECE professional (Institute of Medicine and National Research Council, 2015). These recommendations hold promise for helping to retain highly effective practitioners and expanding access to quality ECE for more young children, including those from diverse socioeconomic status (SES), cultural, and linguistic backgrounds, as well as young children with developmental delays or disabilities.

Recommendation I: Expand Funding Sources and Increase Compensation

The early childhood education (ECE) system has been chronically underfunded in the U.S. for decades. For example, the average spending for ECE in economically developed countries is .7% of the gross domestic product (GDP). In contrast, public spending for ECE in the U.S. funding represents a remarkably small portion of the GDP at less than 0.2% (Learning Policy Institute, 2021). Furthermore, the funding sources are fractured and include federal, state, and local governments, private sector, philanthropic organizations, and out-of-pocket payments. Different funding streams have been initiated with different purposes and have resulted in disparities in quality standards. For example, public schools provide equal access to education, child care subsidies enable adults to work, and Head Start and other pre-K programs were designed to reduce disparities in educational outcomes

(Institute of Medicine and National Research Council, 2015). This diversity in funding and purposes has had negative outcomes for children and professionals. One of the results of a field operating consistently with low and fractured funding is the low pay for a diverse workforce.

Despite the integral role that early childhood educators play, they are compensated with low to poverty wages for their work. Their pay varies by setting; for example, child care workers remain nearly at the bottom of all U.S. occupations when ranked by annual pay; they struggle to make ends meet, frequently relying upon public income support programs. The National Survey of Early Care and Education (NSECE) found that full-time teachers in center-based child care are paid, on average, $14.01 per hour (Datta & Zapata-Gietl, 2023). This results in a yearly wage that often falls under the poverty line. Wages are even lower for infant and toddler classrooms at $10.86 per hour. In contrast, kindergarten teachers in public schools earn double as much as child care teachers. Among those child care teachers who have obtained at least a four-year degree, wages are still far behind their kindergarten counterparts (Datta & Zapata-Gietl, 2023). The Center for the Study of Child Care Employment found that 53 percent of child care workers or their family members were enrolled in at least one public support program, compared with 21 percent of the U.S. workforce as a whole (Coffey, 2022).

Chapter 6 underscores the importance of stable funding, especially in a time of global crisis, and highlights the need to ensure funding reaches the diverse ECE workforce, including HBCC providers. Obtaining affordable child care, such as the lower cost of home-based child care, is often at the expense of lower wages paid to providers (U.S. Department of the Treasury, 2021). Historically lower pay, coupled with pandemic mandates to serve only essential workers and to reduce enrollment, left several ECE educators in precarious financial positions (Center for the Study of Child Care Employment, 2020). Stable funding can ameliorate the negative impacts of crises and secure affordable child care for more families.

Young children learn best when they have positive interactions with adults who are knowledgeable on how to foster learning and cognitive development as well as social and emotional skills (Institute of Medicine and National Research Council, 2015). These interactions are only possible when professionals are respected, trained, and well compensated. Chapter 8 highlights the need for improving the perception, appreciation, and respect for the complex ECE profession. Nevertheless, improving the social standing of ECE professionals is directly tied to improving compensation and qualifications.

Recommendation II: Expand Universal Access and Inclusive Practices

Access to ECE varies greatly in the U.S. based on family income and SES, linguistic background, state of residence, and a child's developmental needs. In most industrialized countries, nearly all children have access to ECE (Organization for Economic Cooperation and Development [OECD], 2019). On average, 87% of 3–5-year-olds in OECD countries enroll in early childhood education. The highest enrollment rates of 3-year-olds in ECE are found in Belgium, Denmark, France, Hungary, Iceland, Israel, Norway, Spain, and the United Kingdom, where they exceed 95% (OECD, 2019). In the last ten years, the average enrollment of 3–5-year-olds in pre-primary education in OECD countries rose from 76% to 87%. This contrasts with trends in the U.S., where less than 54% of 3-and 4 years old participate in any preschool education (Learning Policy Institute, 2021). This varies by state, as some states are making important strides in providing access to preschool. Currently, only five states (Washington, DC, Vermont, Oklahoma, Florida, and Wisconsin) serve 70% of all of their 4-year-old children (Friedman-Krauss et al., 2020).

Universal access is directly tied to cost. There are also many children whose families earn just over the income eligibility threshold to be eligible for publicly funded child care or preschool and yet cannot afford the cost of high-quality ECE - which in many states costs more than college tuition. Expansions in access are directly tied to expansions in funding. For these reasons, there is a need to increase federal support to better match the spending trends in other developed countries. Federal funding can help secure wide access to high quality ECE for all children. Similarly, states should be incentivized to move towards universal preschool programming. Universal programs have the potential to support educational practices for children of diverse SES, linguistic backgrounds, and abilities, and ensure inclusive practices are implemented.

Research shows that inclusive practices in cultural, linguistic, and ability in diverse environments result in a positive effect on children's learning and achievement (Reid et al., 2015). Yet, one of the effects of having a fractionated system with several sources of funding is a lack of inclusivity and diversity in programs. For example, Head Start preschools serve children in poverty, which means that children are unintentionally segregated by SES. Socioeconomic segregation often results in racial, ethnic, and linguistic segregation. Similarly, special education and early intervention programs only serve children with disabilities, and in many cases, they operate in isolation -even when inclusive general education classes might be the best option for students.

High quality ECE has shown to be particularly important for young dual language learners (DLLs). Research shows that children who enter ECE by the age of 3 and remain enrolled longer demonstrate higher language scores and better self-regulation skills. The results have shown to be stronger for DLLs than for monolingual children (Century Foundation, 2020). Chapter 5 described how the pandemic highlighted the challenges immigrant children face and the gap in ECE opportunities for this group. Access to high quality ECE opportunities for children in immigrant families should be a policy priority. The needs are similar for DLLs, as the process of learning a second language in early childhood is difficult and anxiety-provoking. High quality ECE where both English and home language skills are supported play a key role in the later successful transition to official schooling for young DLLs (Plotka & Kim, 2016).

Chapter 6 highlighted the way the existing systems failed children with developmental delays and disabilities during the pandemic, as so many did not receive timely and needed interventions. To extend access for children with disabilities and improve inclusive practices, there is a need to expand new and existing funding streams to secure special education services and evidence-based learning strategies and interventions to meet student needs. For educators to respond to students' social, emotional, and academic needs, as well as use individualized approaches to provide specialized instruction and related services in the least restrictive environment, they need more training. Inclusive practices dictate that all educators become familiar with observation and screening tools, as well as the referral process and the identification of disabilities. Additionally, training educators and implementing trauma-informed practices in all ECE programs can help determine how to support the academic, social, and emotional learning needs of students with disabilities in the aftermath of COVID-19 (Morando-Rhim & Ekin, 2021).

Universal programs have the potential to support inclusive educational practices for all children, including children of diverse SES, linguistic backgrounds, and abilities.

Recommendation III: Establish Standards for High Quality Early Childhood Education

Establishing and enforcing rigorous quality standards for ECE programs can ensure that all children have access to high quality education. Quality standards in the context of ECE refer to a set of guidelines, benchmarks, and criteria that define and ensure high-quality educational experiences for young children. These standards outline expectations for various aspects of ECE programs, including curriculum, teaching practices, health and safety, assessment, professional qualifications, and program administration. Accreditation systems, along with regular monitoring and evaluation, can help maintain and improve uniform expectations for all programs.

At this time, standards vary by state and setting. For example, pre-kindergarten programs in public school districts follow the state educational curricula, while Head Start programs answer to their own set of standards. Standards for child care programs, HBCC, and infant and toddler programs are inconsistent or non-existent. This creates disparate expectations and experiences for children. For example, some children might have spent three years before entering formal schooling in a setting that promotes cognitive development, while others might have spent the same three years watching television most of the day. By the time children enter kindergarten, gaps in educational experiences, skills, and knowledge are often irreversible and follow them through their schooling (García & Weiss, 2015).

High quality developmentally appropriate curriculum is connected across developmental domains and addresses a child's social, emotional, cognitive, language and physical development. Quality early childhood education usually involves an interdisciplinary approach where language and literacy, mathematics, science, and socio-emotional skills are integrated. Developmentally appropriate curriculum exposes children to prerequisite math skills and science inquiry to promote deep understanding of conceptual content and science skills and with language and literacy and socio-emotional competencies always embedded in the curriculum. Detailed and rich connections across domains and subject areas allow for integration of knowledge and skills (National Academies of Science, 2015). For educators to develop a high quality and interdisciplinary curriculum that meets the developmental needs of young children, they need to be highly trained.

At the center of a quality ECE curriculum is the role of play. Chapter 4 explored the challenges experienced when opportunities for play are diminished. The COVID-19 pandemic has highlighted the importance of play for children's cognitive, social, and emotional development, including mental health and well-being (Graber et al., 2021). One of the important lessons learned during these days was the ability for play to reduce play and anxiety and to support emotional growth and resilience (O'Keeffe & McNally, 2021). The growth in awareness of the role of play as a tool for fostering resilience has increased, and this awareness should continue to guide practices in the field. High quality education should not come at the expense of play. Play can foster emotional competencies while facilitating scientific inquiry, language skills, and mathematical thinking. In order to do this effectively, the field needs a qualified and well-paid workforce.

Lastly, parent involvement and engagement are at the cornerstone of high quality early childhood education (Guirguis & Plotka, 2019). Positive communication between educators and families predicts academic motivation, better grades, social skills, and emotional development (McWayne et al., 2004). Additionally, it enhances parent-child and parent-school relationships supporting emotional and behavioral development, self-regulatory skills, and attitudes towards school (De Gaetano, 2007; Cruz, 2016). Chapters 1 and 2 highlight the role of parent communication and support as positive protective factors during the pandemic. Communication is especially important for children with disabilities and DLLs. However, families often face barriers to engagement and communication with educators, and these barriers are often more pronounced for immigrant families. Family engagement is a complex process that requires families to enter a dyadic partnership with their early education educators, and barriers vary from language, cultural, socioeconomic, schedule constraints, immigration status, and feeling unwelcome in the classroom (Moody &

Ramos, 2014). One lesson learned during the pandemic was that family communication and engagement improved when educators used digital tools to connect with families. These achievements gained during these difficult periods should be sustained to expand access and engagement. Future practice should include the incorporation of digital tools for parents to participate in classroom activities, conferences, and meetings. In addition, digital tools should be incorporated to expand both formal and informal communication with parents including the sharing of newsletters and classroom news. These digital tools can also help reduce language barriers and help better reach linguistically diverse families. Reducing barriers to family involvement can help improve the impact of high quality ECE.

Recommendation IV: Develop and Support a Well-Qualified Workforce

Educators need to be highly trained in order to develop and implement high quality inclusive curriculum that addresses a child's social, emotional, language, cognitive, and physical development while integrating literacy, math, science, and other content areas through play. The requirements for early childhood professional and accreditation in the U.S. are not uniform, and often depend more on the ECE setting where adults work rather than on the needs of children (Institute of Medicine and National Research Council, 2015). The differences in licensure requirements for each type of early childhood setting, such as preschool, Head Start, child care and HBCC creates a divide regarding salary and benefits. Aligning qualification requirements across settings and with a set of national standards would create a more equitable pay system (McLean et al., 2021). Well-prepared educators are key to quality early childhood education programs. To date, qualification requirements range from state to state and program to program. For example, in several states, ECE educators must hold a master's degree in the field to qualify for certification and employment as a lead educator. Nevertheless, in many states educators need as much as a high school diploma or equivalent. The United States Department of Health and Human Services (2019) found that among early childhood professionals, 29.9% have a college degree or higher, 17.7% have an associate's degree, 29.62% have some college education but no degree, 19.86% hold a high school degree or equivalent, and 1.69% did not graduate high school. A uniform standard for preparation of professionals is necessary.

Several experts have recommended requiring a minimum expectation of a bachelor's degree for lead early childhood educators, much like the requirements for teachers in formal education settings across the U.S. (Institute of Medicine and National Research Council, 2015). Working with young children requires high levels of sophistication and knowledge, and an understanding of developmentally appropriate practices; it also requires working with children with developmental delays and disabilities, DLLs, and partnering with diverse families. Holding lower education expectations of ECE perpetuates the perception that educating young children requires less expertise than educating older children. This helps justify policies that result in lower funding and lower quality programs, which perpetuates the gap in quality of learning for children from diverse backgrounds (Institute of Medicine and National Research Council, 2015).

Innovative financing strategies will be necessary to help ameliorate the cost of training and higher pay. New preparation standards will require scholarships and stipends for individuals, subsidies for higher education programs, and adjustments to the increased labor costs that will result from higher compensation and benefits for ECE professionals. Financing strategies will be necessary in order to avoid reduced diversity in the professions, increased out-of-pocket costs to families, and increased cost to small child care programs. Lastly, innovative pathways and timelines for individuals will need to be differentiated for currently practicing professionals and prospective educators (Institute of Medicine and National Research Council, 2015).

One way of ensuring more teachers meet their qualifications is making it easier for ECE teachers to become certified by offering some parts of their degrees online. As Chapter 3 shows, higher education students preparing to become early childhood educators appreciate both in-person learning and online options, and most future ECE professionals prefer a combination of both. To facilitate entry into the profession, and the development of a well-prepared highly educated ECE professional, institutions of higher education should develop hybrid models to increase convenience without losing the opportunities for in-person learning. The current trend that started before the pandemic is moving several components of teacher preparation online. In several cases, entire programs have shifted online. The lessons learned during this period should highlight the benefits of multiple modes of instruction with hybrid options and a combination of remote synchronous, asynchronous, and in-person learning to provide maximum flexibility.

Conclusion

COVID-19 brought to light several challenges that were not new to the field of ECE. These challenges existed before the pandemic and will continue to shape the field for years to come. The lessons learned during these dark times should help guide a path forward. For too long, policies for the ECE field have been making do with existing systems instead of focusing on what is needed and committing to strategies necessary to achieve them. Changes should be driven by developmental science and the needs of children, which became clear during this crisis. The recommendations presented in this chapter have the potential for helping train and retain a highly effective workforce, expanding access to quality early childhood education for all young children - including those from diverse SES, cultural, and linguistic backgrounds, and young children with developmental delays or disabilities - while maintaining high standards of developmentally appropriate curriculum.

References

Century Foundation and the Poverty & Race Research Action Council; Children's Equity Project and the Bipartisan Policy Center. (2020). *Expanding inclusive learning for children with disabilities: What we know, what we don't know, and what we should do about it.*

Coffey, M. (2022). (rep.). *Still Underpaid and Unequal.* American Progress: CAP 20. https://www.americanprogress.org/article/still-underpaid-and-unequal/.

Cruz, I. M. (2016, August 1). *Parental involvement: Barriers hispanic parents face.* SUNY Open Access Repository (SOAR). https://soar.suny.edu/handle/20.500.12648/5081.

Datta, R.D. & Zapata-Gietl, C. (2023). Workers in Center-based Early Care and Education Classrooms in 2012 and 2019: Counts and Characteristics. OPRE Report No. 2023-193, Washington DC: Office of Planning, Research, and Evaluation, Administration for Children and Families, U.S. Department of Health and Human Services.

De Gaetano, Y. (2007). The role of culture in engaging Latino parents' involvement in school. *Urban Education, 42*(2), 145–162. https://doi.org/10.1177/0042085906296536

Friedman-Krauss, A. H., Barnett, W. S., Garver, K. A., Hodges, K. S., Weisenfeld, G. G., & Gardiner, B. A. (2020). *The state of preschool 2019.* National Institute for Early Education Research.

García, E., & Weiss, E. (2015, June 17). *Early Education Gaps by Social Class and Race Start U.S. Children Out on Unequal Footing.* A Summary of the Major Findings in Inequalities at the Starting Gate. https://www.epi.org/files/2015/Inequality-Starting-Gate-Summary-of-Findings.pdf

Graber, K.M., Bryne, E.M., Goodacre, E. J., Kirby, N., Kulkarni, K., O'Farrelly, & Ramchandani, P. G. (2021). A rapid review of the impact of quarantine and restricted environments on children's play and the role of play in children's health. *Child Care Health Dev., 47*:143–153. https://doi.org/10.1111/cch.12832

Guirguis, R. & Plotka, R. (2019). Engaging Latino Families in Early Childhood Education Programs: Barriers, Misconceptions, and Recommendation. *Dimensions of Early Childhood Education,* 47 (2), 14-20.

Institute of Medicine and National Research Council. (2015). *Transforming the Workforce for Children Birth Through Age 8: A Unifying Foundation.* Washington, DC: The National Academies Press. https://doi.org/10.17226/19401.

Learning Policy Institute. (2021). *Building a national early childhood education system that works.*

McWayne, C., Hampton, V., Fantuzzo, J., Cohen, H. L., & Sekino, Y. (2004). A Multivariate Examination of Parent Involvement and the Social and Academic Competencies of Urban Kindergarten Children. *Psychology in the Schools, 41*(3), 363–377. https://doi.org/10.1002/pits.10163.

Moody, S & Ramos, M. (2014). Culture counts: engaging Black and Latino parents of young children in family support programs. *Child Trends,* 2-16.

Morando-Rhim L., Ekin S. (2021). How has the pandemic affected students with disabilities? A review of the evidence to date. Center for Reinventing Public Education, University of Wisconsin-Madison. https://www.crpe.org/sites/default/files/final_swd_report_2021.pdf

O'Keeffe, C. & McNally, S. (2021). 'Uncharted territory': teachers' perspectives on play in early childhood classrooms in Ireland during the pandemic, *European Early Childhood Education Research Journal, 29*(1), 79-95. https://doi.10.1080/1350293X.2021.1872668.

Plotka, R. & Kim, S. (2016). Myths and Facts Regarding Second Language Acquisition in Early Childhood: Recommendations for Policymakers, Administrators, and Teachers. *Dimensions in Early Childhood, 44,* 20-27

Reid, J. L., Kagan, S. L., Hilton, M., & Potter, H. (2015). *A better start: Why classroom diversity matters in early education.* The Century Foundation.https://tcf.org/content/commentary/a-better-start-why-classroom-diversity-matters-in-early-education/.

United States Department of Health and Human Services. Administration for Children and Families. Office of Planning, Research and Evaluation, and NSECE Project Team (National Opinion Research Center). National Survey of Early Care and Education (NSECE) Public-Use Files, [United States], 2019. Inter-university Consortium for Political and Social Research [distributor], 2023-11-01. https://doi.org/10.3886/ICPSR37941.v6

Acknowledgements

We would like to give the warmest and most sincere thanks to all the wonderful teachers and families who contributed to the completion of this research.

The illustrators of the cover of this book are Latinx female artists who shared the many challenges they faced during COVID-19; Daniella Kaplan and Katherine Guirguis developed the cover of this book based on their emotional and academic journeys during this unprecedented educational disruption worldwide. We thank them for sharing their stories with us.

We thank our students whose questions inspire us to continue to seek answers and improve our practices.

We would like to acknowledge our outstanding contributors and their research expertise for their collaboration and contribution in Section III: Diverse Experiences in the U.S.

Finally, we would like to acknowledge the New York Association of Public Education (NYAPE), Head Start Dialog, Springer Nature, and the Southern Early Childhood Association for granting us permission to reprint some sections of previously published work by the first authors.

www.ingramcontent.com/pod-product-compliance
Lightning Source LLC
LaVergne TN
LVHW101504200926
848483LV00001B/226